DIVINE
HEALING Sermons

WHITAKER
HOUSE

AIMEE SEMPLE
McPHERSON

DIVINE
HEALING Sermons

WHITAKER
HOUSE

All Scripture quotations are taken from the King James Version of the Holy Bible.

Boldface type in Scripture quotations signifies the emphasis of the author.

DIVINE HEALING SERMONS

ISBN: 978-1-60374-957-2
eBook ISBN: 978-1-60374-981-7
Printed in the United States of America
© 1923, 2014 by Whitaker House

Whitaker House
1030 Hunt Valley Circle
New Kensington, PA 15068
www.whitakerhouse.com

Library of Congress Cataloging-in-Publication Data (Pending)

No part of this book may be reproduced or transmitted in any form or by any means, electronic or mechanical—including photocopying, recording, or by any information storage and retrieval system—without permission in writing from the publisher. Please direct your inquiries to permissionseditor@whitakerhouse.com.

1 2 3 4 5 6 7 8 9 10 11   ᵾᵾ   20 19 18 17 16 15 14

"The Spirit of the Lord is upon me, because he hath anointed me to preach the gospel to the poor; he hath sent me to heal the brokenhearted, to preach deliverance to the captives, and recovering of sight to the blind, to set at liberty them that are bruised, to preach the acceptable year of the Lord."

—Luke 4:18–19

"Go your way, and tell John what things ye have seen and heard; how that the blind see, the lame walk, the lepers are cleansed, the deaf hear, the dead are raised, to the poor the gospel is preached. And blessed is he, whosoever shall not be offended in me."

—Luke 7:22–23

FOREWORD

Nineteen twenty-one was a banner year for evangelist Aimee Semple McPherson. She spent most of it on the road, conducting a series of remarkable evangelistic campaigns that would establish her reputation as the "female Billy Sunday." Wherever she went—Dallas, Denver, St. Louis, San Diego, San Jose—journalists filed essentially the same report: "Never have such scenes been witnessed here." McPherson's plain-folk style warmed the crowds; hearty singing united them; curiosity or faith—or both—held their attention. And the expectation of miracles created a palpable excitement.

In many ways, McPherson seemed one with her audiences, an ordinary woman with problems and longings like their own. But people thronged her meetings because they considered that this ordinary woman possessed decidedly extraordinary confidence in the literal truth of a familiar biblical text: *"Jesus Christ the same yesterday, and to day, and for ever"* (Hebrews 13:8). To McPherson, that meant that in 1921, Jesus could be relied upon to do exactly what He had done when He had lived on earth. She titled one sermon, "Is Jesus Christ the Great 'I Am' or the Great 'I Was'?" She described what she meant by comparing her message to a restaurant menu that listed such biblical options as "know-so salvation," holiness, divine healing, or spiritual power as staples. For hundreds of years, she explained, items like these had been in short supply; some had been eliminated entirely from the menus churches offered. But McPherson offered the full old-time biblical menu to any and all. Her message was at once reassuringly familiar and strikingly different.

She insisted that she prioritized "know-so salvation," but her growing public proved eager to test her assurance of the "sameness" of Jesus by bringing the sick to her for healing.

McPherson had believed in divine healing since her conversion in 1908 and testified to several healings in her own experience, but she did not set out to use prayer for the sick as an evangelistic tool. Then came 1921, a year she began with meetings in San Diego, where crowds of insistent people implored her to pray for their healing. She resisted putting healing front and center, though, and vowed that during the first days of any campaign, she would deliver the familiar revival message of sin, repentance, and salvation. Healing, she thought, was generally "children's bread" (see Matthew 15:26; Mark 7:27)—a promise for those in right relationship with God. In her mind, it should not stand apart from the gospel: it was, in fact, a gospel benefit—a claim she supported by quoting Isaiah 53:5: *"He was wounded for our transgressions…and with his stripes we are healed."*

In January 1921, the San Diego venue that had been rented for the meetings could not accommodate the crowds eager to hear McPherson. Her planned two weeks of meetings became five, and attendance kept climbing. She prayed for the sick at specific services; before long, the numbers forced her to switch from praying for individuals to offering general prayers for healing for all. She concluded the San Diego campaign with two mammoth services in San Diego's landmark Balboa Park. The park's 1,200 acres had been improved for the 1915 Panama-California Exhibition and offered a choice venue for public gatherings. The site included the country's only outdoor pipe organ—73 ranks and 4,518 pipes—and the Spreckels Organ Pavilion. Police estimated that thirty thousand people jammed the 2,400-seat pavilion and environs. Dozens of city pastors flanked McPherson on the stage. McPherson roused the crowd with familiar hymns, preached her sermon, and then began to pray for the sick. With her clergy supporters, she spent six hours moving down the prayer line. Darkness fell before they finished.

Reports from San Diego helped make healing more prominent in McPherson's subsequent crusades, and she found the added personal demands grueling. By the time her itinerary brought her to Denver in June 1921, people were arriving from well beyond the city to benefit from her prayers. A first-page story in the *Denver Post* billed her as a faith healer; a few days later, a picture of "stretcher day" at the McPherson revival covered the width of the first page of the paper. Like it or not, once she agreed to pray publicly for the sick, McPherson could not avoid being cast as a healer. She insisted that she healed no one; only Christ could heal. The public shrugged off such distinctions and demanded more.

After Denver, McPherson moved on to San Jose, where invalids crowded the front section of her tent at every service. McPherson blocked out hours of specific days to pray for the sick. An astute reporter noted that the novelty of healing made it attractive. For her part, McPherson saw no novelty. Rather, she anchored it in the ancient gospel and insisted that her message was 99 percent salvation and 1 percent healing. Yet that point seemed lost in the growing enthusiasm for miracles.

When her audiences clamored to experience the "full gospel" McPherson preached, healing was foremost in many minds. As McPherson's public grew, and she turned her energies to mobilizing her supporters, she settled on a rubric for her message. She would preach the "foursquare gospel." Along with salvation, the baptism with the Holy Spirit, and the return of Christ, healing took its place as one of the four pillars of her evangelistic identity. When she incorporated her movement in 1927, she called it the International Church of the Foursquare Gospel.

McPherson recognized early on that not everyone she prayed for would be healed; but, at the same time, her reading of Hebrews 13:8 and Isaiah 53 obligated her to preach and practice healing. Her own experience captured the paradox she neglected to wrestle with in public. She testified to several healings in early life, but during the 1930s, her health began to fail, and healing eluded her.

She died in California in 1944 at the age of fifty-four. The grassroots hunger for miraculous healings that had contributed to her crowds survived, of course, and within five years, a new generation of healing evangelists, at least one thousand strong, formed a loose association known as the Voice of Healing. They gave a new twist to McPherson's declarations of God's power to heal: in their hands, signs and wonders became evangelistic tools, and miracles loomed ever larger in their view of the Christian life. McPherson had been more modest in her claims but equally confident in her message. Alongside several other women and men of her generation, she encouraged people to believe the Bible literally and entrust their souls and bodies to God's care. She did not forbid medicine; in fact, she relied on it for the last decade of her life, even as she remained convinced that Jesus was her Healer.

Aimee Semple McPherson's sermons on healing echo the early Pentecostal conviction that New Testament Christianity was being restored in the last days. Healing was not a novel curiosity but rather part of the old-time religion at the heart of revival-style Christianity.

—*Edith L. Blumhofer*
Director, Institute for the Study of American Evangelicals,
Wheaton College
Author, *Aimee Semple McPherson: Everybody's Sister*

PREFACE

Unto the sick and the suffering, whose weary, thorn-pierced feet have trod affliction's rugged path; unto the weak who have need of strength; and unto the strong, whose heart would fain be skilled in faith to render support to the weak, this book is lovingly dedicated in the name of Him who gave Himself for us and by whose stripes we are made whole.

Day and night I have but to close these eyes of mine to see again, through misty tears, the drawn, white, pain-blanched faces of the afflicted of my people.

One moment I am weeping for the multitudes shut outside the crowded doors and for the thousands we could never reach, though we toiled day and night. And the next, my face is smiling; mine eyes are made to shine through the tears in remembrance of the thousands who went away skipping, with singing in their hearts—straightened of limb, clear of eye, and strong of faith—to take up again the broken, raveled threads of life and weave upon the loom some brighter, fairer picture of a happy, prayer-filled home wherein the Savior spreads His hands in gentle benediction and reigns supreme upon the altar there.

For the mountains shall depart, and the hills be removed; but my kindness shall not depart from thee, neither shall the covenant of my peace be removed, saith the LORD that hath mercy on thee. O thou afflicted, tossed with tempest, and not comforted, behold, I will lay thy stones with fair colours, *and lay thy foundations with sapphires. And I will make thy windows of agates, and thy gates of carbuncles, and all thy borders of pleasant stones. And all thy children shall be taught of the* LORD; *and great shall be the peace of thy children. In righteousness shalt thou be established: thou shalt be far from oppression; for thou shalt not fear: and from terror; for it shall not come near thee. Behold, they shall surely gather together, but not by me: whosoever shall gather together against thee shall fall for thy sake. Behold, I have created the smith that bloweth the coals in the fire, and that bringeth forth an instrument for his work; and I have created the waster to destroy. No weapon that is formed against thee shall prosper; and every tongue that shall rise against thee in judgment thou shalt condemn. This is the heritage of the servants of the* LORD, *and their righteousness is of me, saith the* LORD.*

(Isaiah 54:10–17)

Should some poor, tempest-driven soul, whose bark is tossed upon the waters of affliction, see shining through these pages the bright and steady light of hope and faith and be guided into the security and calm of the eternal harbor over which the Prince of Peace has spread His healing wings, and should some fellow minister receive new faith and inspiration to go forth and preach the blessed truth of Christ, the Great Physician, whose power is still unchanged and able still to fill the every need of His children (be that need in soul or body)—then I will rejoice indeed, and the glory will be His.

—*Aimee Semple McPherson*

CONTENTS

1. Is Jesus Christ the Great "I Am" or the Great "I Was"?........................15

2. A Double Cure for a Double Curse...25

3. The Scriptural Relationship of Salvation and Divine Healing...........35

4. The Three Parties Concerned in Your Healing....................................43

5. How to Receive Your Healing..55

6. How to Keep Your Healing 69

7. Questions Frequently Asked Regarding Divine Healing 77

8. God's Pattern for a Model Revival 97

9. Some Wonderful Testimonies of Those Healed Through Prayer....107

About the Author 127

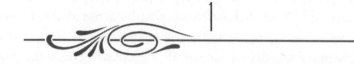

IS JESUS CHRIST
THE GREAT "I AM"
OR THE GREAT "I WAS"?

Shut in my closet of prayer today, with my Bible and the Spirit, my guide, I muse awhile over its pages, then pray for the world with its throngs who, in teeming millions, walk through this life in need of the great I Am.

As I ponder and pray in the stillness, I dream as a dreamer of dreams. A steepled church stands before me—a church with open doors. Within it I see the preacher stand; I hear his voice in earnest call. But it's the throng that flows through the street outside that holds my anxious gaze.

Pit-a-pat! Pit-a-pat!—say the hundreds and thousands of feet surging by the church doors of our land.

Pat! Pat! Pit-a-pat!—hurrying multitudes, bent on business and pleasure.

From out of the church door floats the voice of the pastor and evangelist, in an effort to halt the down-rushing throng in their headlong race toward destruction and to attract their attention to the Christ.

"Stop! Stop, giddy throng, surging by like a river. Take your eyes from the bright lights of the gilded way," they cry. "Leave the paths of death. Enter our open door and listen while we tell you the sweet though ancient story of the great I WAS.

"Eloquently, instructively, we will tell you of the wonderful power Christ *used* to have, the miracles He *used* to perform, the sick He *used* to heal. It's a graphic and blessed history of those things that Jesus did almost nineteen hundred years before you were born. They happened far, far away, across a sea that you have never sailed, in a country that you have never seen, among people you have never known.

"Wonderful, marvelous, was the power that *used* to flow from the great I WAS. He *used* to open the blind eyes, unstop the deaf ears, and make the lame to walk. He *used* to show forth such mighty works, and even manifest them through His followers, that the attention of the multitudes was arrested and gripped in such an irresistible way that thousands were brought storming at His door of mercy to receive blessing and healing at His hand.

"Of course, these mighty works Christ *used* to do are done no longer, for some reason. Perhaps Jesus is too far away or is too busy making intercession at the Father's throne to be bothered with such little things as the physical infirmities of His children. Or His ear may have grown heavy, or His arm be short, or maybe these mighty works were done only to convince the doubters in that day, and since we have no doubters in this civilized day and age, the miraculous has passed away and is no longer necessary.

"At any rate, the fact remains that the signs and wonders that He once declared should accompany His preached Word (see Mark 16) are seen no longer. The power He once displayed, with the glory of His majesty and love coming to destroy the works of the devil, which flashed and played through the gloom like the lightning around Mount Sinai, is now dark, cold, dead. And, as for the visible manifestation of His power, we are left desolate, as though the light that once shone in the darkness had gone out.

"Come, come to this attractive feast, unheeding sinners. Turn now from your Sunday golf, fishing, theaters, and novels. Come enter our doors, that I may tell you the story of the great I WAS and the power that *used* to be."

But—*Pit-a-pat! Pit-a-pat!*—on go the thousands of feet; on to the movie and on to the dance; on to the office, the club, and the bank.

Pat! Pat! Pit-a-pat! "Why don't you stop your wayward feet? Do you not know that you are headed for sorrow? Why is it that the theater is overflowing, while our pews are empty and bare?"

Pat! Pat! Pat! Pit-a-pat! "Oh, stop a moment, the maddening, ceaseless pattering of multitudinous feet, and tell me why you take such interest in the world about you and show such lethargy, carelessness, and lack of active interest in my story of the great I Was and the power He *used* to have and the deeds He *used* to do. Why is it that people grow enthusiastic over the ball game, the boxing ring, the movies, and the dance, while we see no revival of interest or turning to the Christ?"

On and on they go, paying no heed, never turning their eyes from the glittering baubles beyond.

"Why is it, dear Spirit of God," I ask, "they do not listen to that dear brother's call? They do not seem interested in the power Christ *used* to have. In a steady stream they pass by the church and on into the world of grim realities and the problems that they must face."

Pat! Pat! Pit-a-pat!—there are young feet, old feet, light feet, heavy feet, glad feet, sad feet; there are joyous feet and tired, discouraged feet; there are tripping feet and lonely, groping feet; there are straight feet and sick, crippled feet; there are eager, searching feet and disillusioned, disappointed feet. As they pass, a message is somehow tangled up in their pattering, which rises from the cobblestones like a mighty throbbing from the heart of the world.

"'Tis not so much what Christ *used* to do for the world in answer to prayer in bygone days," they seem to say, "but where is His power *now*? And what can He do *today*?"

"Ah, yes!" sigh the crippled feet from the pavement. "We are not so vitally interested in the sick He *used* to heal, the limbs He *used* to make straight and strong. (Of course, we are glad to know that, somewhere, sometime in the distant past, Christ healed the sick in far-off lands.) But we live in the great today, and—*ah me!*—we are very worn and weary! We yearn for healing, hope, and strength today. We stand in need of succor *now*. But you say these mighty provisions for the healing of the body (as well as the soul), which Christ promised in Psalm 103, Isaiah 53, Matthew 8, Mark 16, and James 5, were not at all lasting but were mainly for the Jews who lived in other days. And in reality, your teaching says Christ's healing of the sick, when He walked this earth, was not so much for the demonstration of the tender Savior's love and sake of relieving the sufferers' pain and a pity for the sick themselves as it was to build up His own cause and make the world believe. And when He accomplished this, He withdrew the lifeline of hope and coiled it up again. So, as the church cannot supply my need, I must pass on in further search of help from another source."

"And we," say the tired, discouraged feet, "are also glad that in a far-off land He gave the weary rest, and they, who had well-nigh lost the faith and trust in their fellow man, found truth and grace in Him.

"But you say He is far off now? That we live in a different dispensation? His promises were largely for the Jewish people, anyway? Then there's not much for us here, so we walk past your door, seeking elsewhere a haven of rest and hope."

"And we"—the glad, young, joyous feet send up a rippling echo from the pavement—"we are in search of something that can give us joy and happiness *today*. You say God *used* to make His little ones so happy that they danced and shouted for joy. We, too, want joy! Not the joy that *used* to be but joy of heart *today*. As it is taken away from the church, we seek it in the world."

"And we," say the heavy, groping, lonely feet, "are bereaved and seek comfort and rest. For us, the shades of night are falling. The knowledge that Christ *once* dried tears and bore the heavy load is blest indeed—*but oh!*—we of *today* need help *now*. Preaching the great I WAS can never satisfy our longings; *we need the great I AM*."

The great I AM—why, yes! That's it, exactly! That's what this old world needs: a Christ who lives and loves and answers prayer today, a Christ who changes not (see Malachi 3:6) but is the same *today* as He was yesterday and will be forevermore (see Hebrews 13:8), a Christ whose power knows neither lack nor cessation, a Lord whose name is I AM forever, even unto all generations (see Psalm 146:10).

When the Lord bade Moses to go and call the children of Israel
fleshpots and bondage, the sin and sickness of Egypt, Moses said,

> *Behold, when I come unto the children of Israel, and shall say unto them,*
> *The God of your fathers hath sent me unto you; and they shall say to me,*
> *What is his name? what shall I say unto them? And God said unto Moses,*
> *I AM THAT I AM: and he said, Thus shalt thou say unto the children of*
> *Israel, I AM hath sent me unto you.* (Exodus 3:13–14)

Oh, what a wonderful name! What a wonderful promise. Glory! Glory
to God!

Moses did not need to go about apologetically and say, "The great I WAS
hath sent me unto you. His name is I WAS because He *used* to do great
things—long ago. He expended the last of His power in creating the heavens
and the earth and all that is in them. He is quite far-off now, and the necessity
for this miraculous manifestation of His power is no longer needed, seeing
that all things have now been created. He does not do mighty works today, but
please come and follow and obey the message of the great I WAS."

Why, I doubt whether they would have followed such a call. The message
that Moses bore rang clear and firm—"I AM *hath sent me.*" He walked with
assurance. The solid rock was under his feet. His God was a living God—a
miracle-working God. Moses knew his business was to preach and deliver
the message God had given him. The great I AM had contracted to back up
that message with signs following. "I AM—I AM—I AM!" rang in the ears of
Moses every step he took.

Ah! It gives a servant of God some heart to know that I AM has sent him.
No more apologizing. No more hanging the head and resorting to earthly
means; no more trembling and fear of failure; no dread now that the crowds
will not follow! Head erect, footsteps firm and full of assurance, earthly temple
clad with a robe of the majesty and tenderness of the Father, hands pointing
unhesitatingly to the way, voice ringing clear and authoritative: "I AM...I AM
hath sent me unto you"!

I AM lives today. He will tabernacle in our midst. I AM will deliver us
from our enemies. He will guide us by His hand. I AM will feed us with the

bread from the heavens and give us water from the rock. I Am will deliver us from the sickness and the diseases of the Egyptians, saying, "If you will walk in My ways and keep My statutes, none of the diseases that have been put upon the Egyptians will come near you." I AM will lead us into the Promised Land. (See Exodus 15:26.)

Oh, the blessed assurance, the authority, and the majestic glory of the name I Am! No wonder the children of Israel left the fleshpots and the bondage that hounded them. No wonder the weary eyes of the toiler looked up with new interest and hope. No wonder the hands that hung down were lifted and the feeble knees were made strong when Moses could promise them that when the Lord said to those who were weak, "Be strong and of good courage, for the Lord will do great things" (see Deuteronomy 31:6), He meant just what He said. He did not have to say, "The Lord _used_ to do great things," but could triumphantly declare, "The Lord _will_ do great things, for He is the great I Am, and although heaven is His home, the earth is His footstool, where He answers the prayers of His people."

During Moses' ministry, the sick were healed, the lepers were cleansed, and the plague was stayed.

Oh, Moses, how we envy you the great commission, "Go! Call My people out of bondage into liberty; out of darkness into light; out of sin into holiness; out of sickness into health!" But tell us, just when did the day of supernatural, miraculous manifestation of the power of God end? When did I AM become I WAS?

Why, little children, I AM has never changed! His power is just the same in this day as it was in the days of old. Did He not say, _"This is my name for ever…unto_ **all** _generations"_ (Exodus 3:15)? Those who have faith will see the lightning of His glory flash in power of answered prayer today, as in the days of old. Elijah and Elisha lived in a day when doubters said the miraculous had passed away and I AM had become I WAS. But, through faith and prayer, they proved His name to be I AM to their generations. After the ascension of the only begotten of the Father, Jesus Christ, the disciples proved that He who was dead is alive forevermore (see Revelation 1:18)—the great I AM who saves and heals and baptizes with the Spirit's power.

On and on through the centuries, though surrounded by unbelief and skepticism, there have always been the Elijahs and the Peters who have proved that I Am is His name, even to *their* generations. John Wesley believed that Christ was not only to save but to heal the sick in *his* day. In his biography, he tells of the lame made to walk, of cancers that melted away, and even of a lame horse made whole through answered prayer; thus, he proved I Am to be the Lord's name even to *his* generation.

Then, surely, He has not changed at this late hour! Surely He is the same today. Elijah, Peter, John Wesley, and an army of others who heard and obeyed the message—"*Thus shalt thou say...I Am hath sent me*"—were ridiculed and persecuted by those whom they loved the best. Even so today, although it means being despised and misunderstood, you must get alone in the wilderness of quiet and stillness before God. Seek His face till your soul is kindled with the flame of love from the burning bush. Get your authority from God.

Inquire of Him, "When they ask who sent me, and what is His name, what should I say to them?"

Hear His reply: "*Thus shalt thou say...I Am hath sent me*," and let it ring in your soul forever, louder, clearer, and more wonderful in its revelation of the ever-living Christ with each new step and turn of the way. Victory is assured. The only solution to the problem of drawing the multitude is to lift up not the dead but the *living* Christ; not the great I Was but the great I Am.

Thanks for that message, dear Lord. The clouds of uncertainty are dispelled; the shades of night are rolled back. We see You in a new and glorious light, even as the Son of righteousness with healing in Your wings. (See Malachi 4:2.) I Am is Your name today and will be forever!

I am the Lord, I change not.   (Malachi 3:6)

I [I Am] have redeemed thee, I have called thee by thy name.
                                                                                 (Isaiah 43:1)

I am come down to deliver them...and to bring them up...unto a good land and a large, unto a land flowing with milk and honey.
                                                                                 (Exodus 3:8)

I am [not I WAS but I AM] *the* LORD *that healeth thee.* (Exodus 15:26)

I am He that liveth, and was dead; and, behold, I am alive for evermore.
(Revelation 1:18)

I am Alpha and Omega, the beginning and the end, the first and the last.
(Revelation 22:13)

How the I AMs of the Lord come rolling in, like the billows of a full, over-flowing sea whose tide rises higher toward down-bending heavens.

Glory! Glory! My own poor heart is running over like a tiny cup that would seek to hold the ocean! God is speaking in my ears, "*I AM THAT I AM*" (Exodus 3:14). The earth resounds with His voice. The eternal hills and the mountains swell with the song, "I AM shall be My name forevermore." And away up yonder, the glorious stars of the heaven echo back again: "Even unto all generations, this shall be My name." Angels and cherubim bend low over heaven's balustrade and sing a new song of inspiration: "Go forth, my child, and this your cry will be: '*I AM has sent me unto you.*'"

Again, I see the steepled church, but now the scene is changed.

Pat! Pat! Pit-a-pat!—the street that lies before it is still filled with people. But they are no longer passing by; the crowds are passing in. They fill the pews and the galleries. They stand in the aisles and climb to the windowsills. They pack the doorways and stand on the stairs. The streets and the lanes are filled. The gospel nets are full to bursting, and there is no more room to contain the multitudes that throng the place.

And out over the heads of the people, I hear the message ring:

"Awake, you who sleep, and arise from the dead! The Lord still lives today. His power has never abated. His Word has never changed. The things He did in Bible days, He still lives to do today. There is no burden He cannot bear, nor fetter He cannot break.

"Here, bring your sins; He'll wash them away. Here, bring your sicknesses; He'll heal you today. We serve not a dead but a *living* God—not I WAS, but the great I AM.

"Come young, come old; come sad, come glad; come weary and faltering of step; come sick, come well; come one, come all, unto the great I Am. There is food for the hungry; there is strength for the faint; there is hope for the hopeless and sight for the blind."

Pit-a-pat! Pit-a-pat! Faster and faster they come! The church is overflowing; they are filling the streets. Their faces are shining; in their eyes, the light of hope has been kindled by the taper of faith through the preaching of the great I Am.

They are reaching out their hands for forgiveness, for the healing of the crippled and sick. They are thirsting for the joy of salvation and hungering for the Bread of Life. They are seeking the power of the Holy Spirit and something practical that can meet the immediate and pressing need of the great today and prepare them for tomorrow. And they have found the source of sure supply *in the church*—the house of God—from under whose altar and over whose threshold runs the ever-deepening stream of life. They seek no farther through the briers of the world; they have found the great I Am, and they sing:

> Wisdom, righteousness and pow'r,
> Holiness forevermore,
> My redemption full and sure,
> He is all I need.[1]

Burdens are lifted; tearful and weeping eyes are dried; the sick are healed; the crooked are made straight. Sin-guilty hearts are cleansed and made holy. Empty water pots are filled with wine. And the cold, worldly church has risen from the dust in garments that are glistening and white. With oil in their lamps and sheaves in their arms, they worship the great I Am.

---

1. Charles P. Jones, "He Is All I Need," 1906.

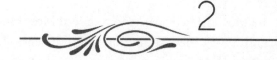

2

A DOUBLE CURE FOR
A DOUBLE CURSE

When Satan entered the purity of the garden of Eden in the form of a serpent, two angels of darkness followed hard on his trail. His coming brought the double curse of sin and sickness.

When Christ came into the dying world to redeem it from the curse, there came in His blessed footsteps two angels of light and hope. His coming brought the double cure: salvation and healing.

In the beginning, the world emerged from under the hand of God, good and pure and perfect. In the garden of Eden, the most perfect spot in a perfect world, He placed the perfect man and woman, Adam and Eve, whom He had formed from the dust of the ground and into whose nostrils He had breathed the breath of life.

In innocence and purity, they dwelled beneath the flowing boughs and trailing flowers of rich, fruit-laden trees. Busy bees droned contentedly in the perfumed air as the golden, mellow sunlight of a perfect day filtered through the dense green foliage of leaf and branch and splashed upon a floor carpeted with violets, moss, and lichen. Birds of rich plumage flitted from tree to tree, and high above it all, a songful lark sprang into the open heaven, showering the air with musical praise.

Into the tranquil beauty of this garden, which His own loving hand had planted, God loved to walk in the cool of the day, communing with man, whom He had made after His own image and filled with His breath divine.

How peaceful their abode! How blessed their communion! How blissful their freedom of body, soul, and spirit! They had but one requirement—faith in the Word of the Father and obedience to His command.

But alas! The gleaming, malevolent, calculating eyes of Satan were watching from the distance, with seething hatred for God and jealousy of man fermenting in his soul and cunning planning in his heart. Once, he had been an angel of authority in heaven, but because of jealousy, disobedience, and treachery, he had fallen as a flaming torch from heaven, drawing a third of the angels with him. (See Luke 10:18; Isaiah 14:12–14.)

The burning passion in his diabolic nature now longed for revenge—for a way to strike back. And here—here in this blissful garden of Eden, with its stately trees, its hanging flowers, its luscious fruitage, and its dancing, sparkling brooks and rivers, where God had placed the children of His own dear handiwork—he had found the place for revenge!

Now who did the Father so love as these children? Had He not toiled through the days to create the earth for his habitation? And what was there in heaven or on earth that so grieved and pierced the pure heart of the Father as disobedience and sin? Has it not been written that: God cannot look upon sin with the least degree of allowance? Has He not said: *"The soul that sinneth, it shall die"* (Ezekiel 18:20)? Full well did Satan know that God, in His justice, would show no partiality. And though His heart was torn and bleeding, the curse of His disapproval must fall upon the inmates of the garden, and the whole earth must be jolted and shaken with the impact of the fall.

With fiendish cunning, Satan took upon himself the form of a flashing, scintillating serpent (said at that time to be the most beautiful and subtle beast of the field), and in shimmering, graceful strides and his most captivating manner, he drew near to the woman and began to sow the fateful seeds of unbelief within her heart:

But of the fruit of the tree which is in the midst of the garden, God hath said, Ye shall not eat of it, neither shall ye touch it, lest ye die. And the serpent said unto the woman, Ye shall not surely die. (Genesis 3:3–4)

The first lie the devil told the human family, the first seed of doubt he sowed in their hearts, was that of doubting the veracity and absolute, unchangeable truth of God's Word. He has been engaged with the same task ever since.

Behind the devil, as he enters the garden, stand two fearsome demons of night. Our hearts are repulsed and shuddering as we gaze on each cruel face.

Oh, Mother Eve! Could you not see them? Why were your eyes so blinded? On each shield, with which they cover themselves, is the form of a venomous serpent with a parting, darting, poisonous tongue. In his hand, each demon holds a fork with sharp, barbed prongs, with which to pierce body and soul with fearful wounds that no earthly power can heal. Oh, Eve! Can't you see them, hand in hand, an invincible, inseparable pair—twin angels of darkness, agents of despair, relentless and cruel? Their names are written on their shields: Sin and Sickness.

But the eyes of Eve were riveted in fascination on the shimmering serpent's form! Her ears hearkened to that smooth deceiver's voice. Thus Eve was deceived, and in obeying the word of Satan, she disobeyed her Lord, ate of the forbidden fruit, and gave Adam to eat also.

Soon came the footsteps of God, walking in the garden in the cool of the evening. "Adam, where art thou?" His voice rang out in tones of thunder that struck fear and quaking into those guilty souls who sought to hide from His gaze. Quick as a flash, His keen, all-seeing eye read the story, and His heart was grieved and sad. They had sold themselves to the devil, and the twin demons of darkness laughed as they reached out through the gathering gloom, the more firmly to grip the erring ones on the prongs of suffering and sin.

Hand in hand came sin and sickness into the garden of life. Hand in hand they have walked through the years since that day. But instead of leaving His children in the hands of the devil to suffer the double curse they had brought upon themselves through disobedience, the great, loving Father heart of God began even then to lay plans for their redemption—a double cure for a double curse.

But there and then, even though man had to be driven from the garden, God gave His first prophetic promise, that through the seed of woman would come Him who would bruise the head that bruised His heel. All down through the coming years that led by a winding trail, through many lands and many tears, on through the days of Abel, Seth, Noah, Shem, Abraham, Isaac, Jacob, Judah, and David—even down to the cross of Christ—this promise was reiterated through the prophets and sages.

Thus it was that, as far back as the days of Moses, it was an understood fact that salvation and healing were provided in the atonement through the Lamb slain from the foundation of the world. When Moses brought the children of Israel from Egypt and turned their faces toward the Promised Land, God spoke to them, saying:

> *If thou wilt diligently hearken to the voice of the* Lord *thy God, and wilt do that which is right in his sight, and wilt give ear to his commandments, and keep all his statutes, I will put none of these diseases upon thee, which I have brought upon the Egyptians: for I am the* Lord *that healeth thee.*
> (Exodus 15:26)

Clearly the Father signified that with disobedience and sin would come sickness and disease. Later, when disobedience and sin had laid them low, and fiery serpents bit them till they died, God commanded that a brazen serpent (brass signifying judgment) should be lifted up in the wilderness, even as Christ was later to pass through the judgment for us and be lifted up on the cross of Calvary. Those who looked upon the serpent that was lifted up in the wilderness had life for a look. They found therein the double cure—forgiveness for the soul and healing for the body.

When Miriam, through the sin of criticism and backbiting, fell ill of leprosy white as snow, Moses besought God for the double cure. After pleading the mercy and pardon of the Lord, he cried, *"Heal her now, O God, I beseech thee"* (Numbers 12:13).

Of the double cure for the double curse, the psalmist spoke clearly, saying, *"Bless the* Lord, *O my soul, and forget not all his benefits: who forgiveth all thine iniquities; who healeth all thy diseases"* (Psalm 103:2–3). Notice that the first two benefits David mentions are those of forgiveness and salvation, which overthrow the powers of sin, and divine healing for the body, which overthrows sickness and disease.

Isaiah, catching sight of the great Redeemer through the lifted veil, beheld Christ as the Man of Sorrows and acquainted with grief. He saw in His glorious coming the double cure for the double curse and declared of His work of atonement, *"He was wounded for our transgressions, he was bruised for our iniquities* [notice the word *"bruised"*—God had said of Him that He would bruise the head that bruised His heel]...*and with his stripes we are healed"* (Isaiah 53:5).

"Does not this promise refer to spiritual healing only?" asks one timid soul to whom the news seems almost too good to be true. No, Matthew 8:16–17 describes Christ healing the sick, casting out demons, and causing the blind to see and the lame to walk, and then it tells us that this physical healing is the literal interpretation of Isaiah 53. In verse 17, Matthew noted that this was done *"that it might be fulfilled which was spoken by Esaias the prophet, saying, Himself took our infirmities, and bare our sicknesses."*

The coming of Jesus Christ, the Son of God, the seed of woman, was the coming of the great deliverer to redeem a stricken world from the curse. Speaking of His own mission, Jesus plainly said,

> *The Spirit of the Lord is upon me, because he hath anointed me to preach the gospel to the poor; he hath sent me to heal the brokenhearted, to preach deliverance to the captives, and recovering of sight to the blind, to set at liberty them that are bruised, to preach the acceptable year of the Lord.*
> (Luke 4:18–19)

O blessed Light that shines in the darkness, even though the darkness comprehends it not! O blessed Burden-Bearer, who carries our sins, bears our sicknesses, and endures our pain—would that the world might see You!

Oh, look, heart-sore world, can't you see the two great blessings that follow the Master wherever He goes, like two bright angels of light, who stand, hand in hand, with shining swords bearing the sign of the cross and holding aloft the Spirit's sword to cut your bonds in two? Salvation declares, *"Thy sins be forgiven thee"* (Mark 2:5). Healing cries, *"Arise, and take up thy bed, and walk"* (Mark 2:9). And over mountain and dale, in valley or plain, within the palace and in the hut—wherever this dear Jesus of Galilee went—He brought with Him this double cure, salvation and healing.

"*Wherefore think ye evil in your hearts?*" said He. "*For whether is easier, to say, Thy sins be forgiven thee; or to say, Arise, and walk?*" (Matthew 9:4–5). Which is easier? Who is there among us who would dare to say? For this heaven-horn, heaven-sent pair stands hand in hand, shield to shield—a double cure for a double curse. In God's plan, they should never be divided.

When the short years of our Lord's ministry, wherein He went about destroying the works of the devil—namely, forgiving sin and healing the sick—were ended, the hour approached for His torturous death on the cross. Emerging from Gethsemane Garden when the long night was over, He was condemned before Pontius Pilate to die on the rugged tree.

But before they led Him up Calvary's mountain, something of great importance needed to take place—something that makes our cheeks blanch and our teardrops start at the very thought. They needed to bare our Savior's back to the smiters, tie Him to the whipping post, and flog Him with the cruel lash.

Did you ever wonder why?

Blow upon blow fell on the tender, quivering flesh of the gentle Nazarene. The biting whip rose and fell again and again in the hands of the Roman soldier, till the great purple welts stood on the precious back that was so soon to bear the cross—till the drops of blood dripped upon the ground. Some forty blows were permissible in those days, and men often fainted or even died at the whipping post.

"Tell me, dear Spirit, teacher and guide, O tell me, *why* did they whip Him so? Was He whipped that my many sins might be washed away?"

"No, child; the blood on the cross was sufficient for that."

"Then why did they pluck the beard from His face and beat Him with cruel staves? Was that for the cleansing of sin?"

"No, child; the blood was sufficient for that."

"Then why, O Spirit of God, tell me, why did they torture my Savior so? Was God merely permitting the vindictive, fiendish wrath of an angry mob to be wreaked upon the head of His blessed Son? Else if His stripes did not cleanse me from sin, then *why* did they whip Him so?"

"Why, child? Do you not know the meaning of that lash, the cruel blows of the smiters' scourge? It was thus He bore your suffering, and by His stripes you are healed. Not a meaningless blow, not a meaningless pain, did that precious body bear. At the whipping post, He purchased your healing; He bore your suffering and pain. On the cross, He purchased your pardon, forgiveness, and cleansing from sin. You are healed by His stripes, cleansed by His blood—O blessed double cure for a double curse for all who will look and live."

But have not these two been separated, till only salvation remains? Then His stripes were born in vain. Hearken to the words of the Master:

All power is given unto me in heaven and in earth. Go ye therefore, and teach all nations, baptizing them in the name of the Father, and of the Son, and of the Holy Ghost: teaching them to observe all things whatsoever I have commanded you: and, lo, I am with you alway, even unto the end of the world. Amen. (Matthew 28:18–20)

And as ye go, preach, saying, The kingdom of heaven is at hand. Heal the sick, cleanse the lepers, raise the dead, cast out devils: freely ye have received, freely give. (Matthew 10:7–8)

And He sent them to preach the gospel and heal the sick. And He said,

And these signs shall follow them that believe; In my name shall they cast out devils; they shall speak with new tongues; they shall take up serpents; and if they drink any deadly thing, it shall not hurt them; they shall lay hands on the sick, and they shall recover. (Mark 16:17–18)

Jesus—the same yesterday, today, and forever—still brings the double cure for soul and body. There is still life for a look at the crucified One, and those who touch the hem of His garment may still be made whole.

In James 5, the elders of the church are given instructions to anoint the sick (who call for them) with oil and to pray the prayer of faith, having the promise of the double cure.

And the prayer of faith shall save the sick, and the Lord shall raise him up; and if he have committed sins, they shall be forgiven him. Confess your faults one to another, and pray one for another, that ye may be healed.
(James 5:15–16)

What a sweet relationship exists between salvation and healing.

This does not mean that we will never die. There comes a day when the sands of the years are run out, and the child of God is caught up and goes sweeping home to glory. Thank God for that hope! It is not that those who claim the promise of healing fear death; to be absent from the body is to be present with the Lord. (See 2 Corinthians 5:8.) But it does mean that, instead of suffering and groaning all the days of our lives with a torturous disease, it is possible to look to Jesus and take what He paid for with cruel stripes and the shedding of His precious blood.

Too long have we wandered in weakness and poverty, when we might have had His strength and riches! Too long have we lain starving, when we might have been feasting in Father's banquet hall.

A man in strained financial circumstances once bought a ticket for an ocean voyage.

"Now I must be very careful of saving my few remaining dollars," he told himself. "I'll just buy some crackers and drink water with them for the duration of my voyage, thus leaving a small sum for my arrival."

Days wore by, one by one, and the poor man became more and more famished for a good square meal and more disgusted with crackers and water. On the day that the steamer was scheduled to arrive in port, he could bear it no longer. Even if it took the last cent, he decided that he must have one more good meal.

But when he made his way to the dining salon, its beauty and the fine food that was being served—course after course at the tables, with white linen and shining silver—caused him to doubt. Such a fine dining room—perhaps he would not have money enough, after all! Catching the eye of the steward, he inquired, "Sir, would you please be kind enough to tell me the cost of a meal in that dining room?"

The waiter looked at the man with amazement and said, "Why, I don't understand what you mean."

"I want to know how much one good, square meal at that table would cost me, please."

"Why, you have a ticket for this steamship voyage, haven't you?"

"Ticket? Why, y-yes," stammered the man.

"Then your meals don't cost you a penny. They are all included in your ticket. Where have you been at mealtimes? Why did you not come to the table? Your place has been set and held vacant for you all the time."

"Why, I've been sitting in my stateroom, eating crackers and drinking cold water, every day, because I thought I could not afford the dining room."

And, dear ones, many of us have gone almost to the end of life's voyage before realizing the good things included in our ticket. Salvation, healing, the power of the Holy Spirit, and rich life in Christ are yours for the asking. Draw near today and cry, "Son of David, have mercy upon me. I now appropriate Your promises and claim as mine the rich provision You have made for me, even the double cure, with its blessings for body and soul."

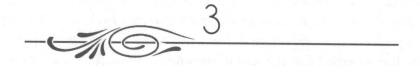

THE SCRIPTURAL RELATIONSHIP OF SALVATION AND DIVINE HEALING

In God's great plan of redemption, salvation for the soul and divine healing for the body were united in holy matrimony and destined to walk together, hand in hand, through the ages. Unbelief has sought to divorce this heaven-born pair, but prayer and faith still prove they are united.

Healing for the body was included in the atonement made by Jesus Christ, the Son of God. Beaten with cruel stripes, He purchased healing for the body. Wounded for our transgressions, He bought redemption for every soul who would believe in Him with the whole heart.

In the Beginning

In the beginning, man, through disobedience, transgressed the law of God. Believing the words of Satan rather than the words of God, the inmates of the garden did exactly what God told them not to do, and through their disobedience, they opened the door to that inseparable pair: sin and suffering.

Man sold himself for nothing and engaged himself to be the bond-servant of the devil. Banished from the garden, sweating through the toil of the day, groaning in labor and pain—how hopeless was his state!

But, hark! The voice of God spoke to the man and the woman, and with His promise came a shaft of light from the Son of Righteousness, falling in the midst of the darkness of the night, cleaving it asunder, and promising the opening of a new and living way; spelling deliverance from sin and its awful consequences and the regaining of that which they had lost. For His unfailing Word had promised that the seed of the woman would come and bruise the head that had bruised His heel. Hallelujah!

Through the centuries of the Old Testament, the faithful received forgiveness of their sins and healing for their bodies by believing in Him who would come and bear their grief in His own body on the tree. And thus it was, though plagues were rampant all about them, that the Lord said,

If thou wilt diligently hearken to the voice of the LORD thy God, and wilt do that which is right in his sight, and wilt give ear to his commandments, and keep all his statutes, I will put none of these diseases upon thee, which I have brought upon the Egyptians: for I am the LORD that healeth thee.
(Exodus 15:26)

In Moses' Day

When Miriam fell ill of leprosy because of criticism and backbiting, repentance and faith in the Lord brought forgiveness and healing. The cry *"Alas, my lord…we have done foolishly…we have sinned.…Heal her now, O God, I beseech thee"* (Numbers 12:11–13) brought the answer down from heaven. Forgiveness and healing came forth together to reign in the stead of sickness and sin.

When the children of Israel committed a grievous sin before the Lord, sickness and plague followed hard on its trail, till they died and fell in heaps.

And Moses said unto Aaron, Take a censer, and put fire therein from off the altar, and put on incense, and go quickly unto the congregation, and

make an atonement for them: for there is wrath gone out from the LORD; *the plague is begun. And Aaron took as Moses commanded, and ran into the midst of the congregation; and, behold, the plague was begun among the people: and he put on incense, and made an atonement for the people. And he stood between the dead and the living; and the plague was stayed.*

(Numbers 16:46–48)

Again, sickness and suffering followed the offspring of the devil—sin. And again, salvation and healing followed repentance, obedience, and faith.

And when, through disobedience and sin, they lay dying from the bites of fiery serpents, pardon and healing came together. From the depths of repentance and sorrow, they cried,

We have sinned, for we have spoken against the LORD, *and against thee; pray unto the* LORD, *that he take away the serpents from us. And Moses prayed for the people. And the* LORD *said unto Moses, Make thee a fiery serpent, and set it upon a pole: and it shall come to pass, that every one that is bitten, when he looketh upon it, shall live. And Moses made a serpent of brass, and put it upon a pole, and it came to pass, that if a serpent had bitten any man, when he beheld the serpent of brass, he lived.*

(Numbers 21:7–9)

And to our own hearts, the blessed hope is born, for as the serpent was lifted up in the wilderness, so Christ was lifted up on the cross, bearing our sin, carrying our sorrow, cruelly smitten, and bearing the stripes for our healing.

When the angel of death was passing over Egypt, the children of Israel found peace and safety through the slain Paschal lamb. The broken body of the lamb provided food and strength for their bodily needs, while the blood on the doorpost procured their deliverance and protection. And so it is with Jesus, the Lamb slain from the foundation of the world. Through the stripes and sufferings that He bore, He brings us healing, and His precious blood, upon the lintels of our hearts, brings pardon and the passing over of the wrath of God.

In the Day of David and Isaiah

On and on through the pages of the Word walk salvation and healing side by side. On they walk through David's day; and, seeing them, the psalmist caught up his harp and sang, in a rapturous thanksgiving,

Bless the LORD, O my soul, and forget not all his benefits: who forgiveth all thine iniquities; who healeth all thy diseases: who redeemeth thy life from destruction, who crowneth thee with loving kindness and tender mercies; who satisfieth thy mouth with good things; so that thy youth is renewed like the eagle's. (Psalm 103:2–5)

Our dear, precious Redeemer—with every turned page, His coming is nearer and clearer, till Isaiah 53. And, beholding Him through tear-dimmed eyes of faith, the prophet cried, *"He was wounded for our transgressions…and with his stripes we are healed"* (verse 5).

Everywhere, confident, undisputed, and cooperative relationship and unity are found existing between the salvation of the soul and the healing of the body, which our Redeemer purchased on the cross for all who would *believe with the whole heart.*

In Jesus' Day

With the coming of the Lord, the two were even more visibly and inseparably bound together. He came to destroy the works of the devil (see 1 John 3:8), and through His years of ministry upon the earth, our Lord went about forgiving sin and healing all who were oppressed by the devil. With this sweet and gracious benediction, His words fell upon the troubled heart: *"Neither do I condemn thee: go, and sin no more"* (John 8:11) or, *"Thy sins be forgiven thee… arise, take up thy bed, and go"* (Matthew 9:2, 6). Hallelujah! What a Deliverer is this—what a precious double cure for soul and body! Praise the Lord!

In Matthew 9, a man was brought to Jesus who was sick with palsy and lying on a bed. Jesus, seeing the faith of his friends, said unto the man who was sick with the palsy: *"Son, be of good cheer; thy sins be forgiven thee"* (Matthew 9:2). But, behold, certain scribes, although forced by what their eyes had seen in the past to believe Christ's power to heal the sick, doubted in their hearts His ability to forgive sin. Jesus, knowing their thoughts, said, *"Wherefore think ye evil in your hearts, for is it easier to say, Thy sins be forgiven thee; or to say, Arise, and walk?"* (Matthew 9:5–6).

The scribes of that day had admitted Christ's power to heal but disputed His power to forgive. Today, the attitude of the doubter is quite reversed—some admit His power to forgive sin but doubt His ability to heal the sick. But Jesus says, *"Which is easier?"* And the simple fact is that it is just as easy for the Lord to do the one as the other.

Salvation and Healing—Hand in Hand in the Great Commission

When sending forth His disciples in Matthew 10:7–8, the Lord commanded them, saying, *"As ye go, preach, saying, The kingdom of heaven is at hand. Heal the sick, cleanse the lepers…freely ye have received, freely give."* In His great worldwide commission, under which we live and work for Christ today, Jesus said:

> Go ye into all the world, and preach the gospel to every creature. He that believeth and is baptized shall be saved; but he that believeth not shall be damned. And these signs shall follow them that believe; In my name shall they cast out devils; they shall speak with new tongues…they shall lay hands on the sick, and they shall recover.   (Mark 16:15–18)

Not once is there an intimation that salvation and healing are to be separated. Rather, we hear only the constant assurance that Jesus is the very same yesterday, today, and forever, and His promise that *"He that believeth on me, the works that I do shall he do also; and greater works than these shall he do; because I go unto my Father"* (John 14:12).

In the Acts of the Apostles

In the Acts of the Apostles, divine healing is still the handmaiden of the gospel. *"And they went forth, and preached everywhere, the Lord working with them, and confirming the word with signs following"* (Mark 16:20). The healing of the lame man in Acts 3 resulted in the conversion of five thousand men in Acts 4:4.

When surrounded by the hosts of darkness, unbelief, and fierce opposition, the prayer of New Testament believers was that healing for the body might be the advance guard of faith in the spoken Word:

> *And now, Lord, behold their threatenings; and grant unto thy servants, that with all boldness they may speak thy word, by* [note the connection between the two] *stretching forth thine hand to heal; and that signs and wonders may be done by the name of thy holy child Jesus.*
>
> (Acts 4:29–30)

In Acts 5:12–16, salvation and divine healing are so closely interwoven as to seem almost inseparable.

> *And by the hands of the apostles were many signs and wonders wrought among the people…and believers were the more added to the Lord, multitudes both of men and women. Insomuch that they brought forth the sick into the streets and laid them on beds and couches, that at the least the shadow of Peter passing by might overshadow some of them. There came also a multitude out of the cities round about unto Jerusalem, bringing sick folks, and them which were vexed with unclean spirits: and they were healed every one.*

On and on the apostles journeyed together, to the last chapter of Acts, where Paul, on the Isle of Melita, healed the sick in Jesus' name as freely as he preached the glorious gospel.

According to James

In James 5:14–15, salvation and healing are still united. In the apostle's instructions to the church and the tribes scattered abroad, we read,

Is any sick among you? Let him call for the elders of the church; and let them pray over him, anointing him with oil in the name of the Lord: and the prayer of faith shall save the sick, and the Lord shall raise him up; and [note the connection] *if he have committed sins, they shall be forgiven him.*

What a close harmony exists between salvation and healing! Who would dare cross out the forgiveness and leave the healing, or cross out the healing and leave the forgiveness?

Note the sweet union in the next verse also: *"Confess your faults one to another, and pray one for another, that ye may be healed"* (James 5:16).

And now, God's Word still stands as sure and true as ever. Not one of His good promises has ever crumbled in the dust. Those who come to Christ in full surrender, forsaking the world and seeking Him with all their hearts, in faith and obedience, still find His power the very same.

On Calvary's cross, the great Redeemer carried not only our sin, but *"himself took our infirmities, and bare our sicknesses"* (Matthew 8:17). While many stand in doubt, thinking that His healing power has been withdrawn and that His saving grace alone remains, thousands are laying hold of the promise, taking Christ at His word, and being healed of their diseases.

Oh, the wonderful miracles that our eyes have beheld in the past few months—the blind receiving sight; the deaf ears unstopped; the lame and paralyzed standing and leaping for joy! And how these miracles have brought the sinner weeping to the cross! Hard, sneering skeptics have turned pale and fallen to their knees. Proud women have sobbed and given their hearts to Christ; and, oh, we *know* that Christ is just the same today as in the days of old.

His saving and His healing power are just the same if only we *believe.* While some content themselves with telling only what Christ used to do in days gone by, others are rising up and pressing through the throng to touch His garment now. And by their faith, they are made whole. What a blessed privilege! What a real and practical gospel of power that cannot be denied! What a wonderful Savior is the Christ, who forgives all your iniquities and who heals all your diseases.

4

THE THREE PARTIES CONCERNED IN YOUR HEALING

There are three parties concerned in your divine healing—you, the Lord Jesus, and the one who prays for you. Let us consider just what part each must take in order to bring about your healing. The first to be concerned in your healing is, of course, you.

You

If you want be cleansed and made completely whole, you have a part to do in pressing through the thronging doubt, hindrances, and materialism of the day and touching the hem of the Master's robe. So often, people come to me for prayer who have only a passive faith and are dumbly *hoping* that I can heal them or do all the interceding on their behalf. Though the hands of everyone about them may be lifted in intercession, their faces wet with tears, and a real prayer of faith in their hearts, such ones stand passively—without any real soul outcry to God, waiting for our prayers to heal them and *hoping* it will be done. If they are healed, they will be grateful to those who prayed and say that they *certainly had some kind of power.* If not healed, they will go out and criticize the meeting, telling the people that they *tried it* or *had a treatment* but that it did them no good.

But do you not see that people like this have not done their part in pressing through to Jesus with active faith and believing prayer? You can *try* doctors, *try* medicine, *try* science, *try* baths and electric treatment, but you cannot *try* Jesus Christ. Remember also that neither Christ nor His servants who pray for you give "treatments." That word belongs to doctors or to Christian Science but has no place in the Bible or in these revival meetings. The very fact that one uses this word in this connection would indicate that his heart is far from God and that the truth concerning the atonement and power of the slain Lamb of Calvary is not in him.

The one coming for healing has a real, definite part to play in his coming to the Great Physician.

The disciples had to come to land before they could be warmed at the fire that Jesus had kindled or partake of the fish He had broiled. They had to leave their ship, come to shore, and draw near to Jesus before they could receive the bounties from His hand. You, too, must come out of the ship in which you have gone "fishing" for worldly joys and gains, toiling through the night and catching nothing. Let down your nets on the right side; prove the bounty of His goodness, love, and power; and then jump overboard, like Peter, when his Master bade him, "Come and dine." (See John 21:3–12.)

The prodigal son had to come home before he could receive the kiss of reconciliation, the ring, the best robe, and the shoes for his weary wandering feet. The father could not carry the best robe to his son when he sat among the swine, eating the husks that they did eat. The father could not meet the son on the ground of his prodigality; the son had to return to his father's home and meet him on his own just and righteous ground. Besides, the best robe would soon have been soiled and besmirched, discrediting his father's name, had it been worn in the midst of his reveling and merrymaking. (See Luke 15:11–24.)

Just so, if you want to be made whole and receive the best robe and gifts the heavenly Father has to give—salvation, healing, and the baptism of the Holy Spirit, through the Lord Jesus Christ—you, too, must do your part, leave the land of sin and backsliding (your soul is sick of it all, anyway), and say, "I will arise and go." Come, crying, "Father, I have sinned against heaven and in Your sight." Through the mist of penitent tears, you will surely see the Father running to meet you with clothing, with food, and with gladness. Just as the ring that the father gave the son had no ending but was a complete circle, so the love, promises, and provision of Christ are unending, for He is the same today as He was yesterday and as He will be evermore.

Naaman had to dip seven times in the Jordan before he was cleansed of his leprosy. He had his part to play in obedience and humility. Had Naaman failed to do his part, God could not have done His, and he would have gone away uncleansed. Naaman did not go part of the way to the Jordan but all the way; he dipped not three or four but seven times. If he dipped the first two or three times with the thought of a *treatment* in his mind, the thought was surely washed away before he went down the seventh time in obedience and faith, for he came up every bit whole. (See 2 Kings 5:1–14.)

Many come for healing today just like Naaman went to Elisha. They think they can sit outside in their chariot or automobile and have God's servant run out and heal them. No, no! Rich or poor, bond or free, all must go the same humble road to the Jordan. It is not the servant but the Master who has the power.

The importance of the work of preparation cannot be spoken of too highly or be too greatly emphasized.

People who come blindly, rushing into the meetings, saying that they have heard "there is a miracle woman here who can heal them at once" and that they want to be *treated* at once so they can catch the next train for business and pleasure are quickly disillusioned. First of all, they are informed that there is no "miracle woman" here at all, only a simple little body whom the Lord has called from a milk-pail on a Canadian farm, bidding her to tell the good news of a Savior who lives and loves and answers prayers.

Then they are told to settle themselves down and take part in the meetings, just as though they were going to any great hospital for an operation and were preparing for it for days, obeying each order. So they are hold to prepare their house before coming into the presence of Jesus, the Great Physician. They are reminded that if they rush into a hospital, dirty and dusty and travel-stained, demanding that a serious, major operation should be performed that instant, in order that they might catch the next train for home, the doctors would explain to them that they were in no condition to go to the table as they were, lest infection should set in and their latter condition be more serious than the former.

How clean and purged their systems must be before going to the operating table! Then, how clean and pure their hearts and lives must be before coming to ask the sacred and holy touch of Christ upon their mortal bodies.

How clean the nurse would bathe them—how sterile and white the robe she would dress them in before they were wheeled to the operating table! How pure, then, they must be, spiritually washed in the blood of Jesus and clad in the white robes of righteousness, beneath which heart and life and soul are made pleasing in His sight, before coming for healing.

The results of this preparation are self-evident. They are wonderful. Cancers have disappeared, fibroid tumors have melted like snow before the sun, goiters have gone down like a toy balloon that is punctured, stiff limbs have been made to bend, blind eyes have recovered sight, deaf ears have been unstopped, dumb lips have been opened, and withered arms have come to life and grown several inches in an hour.

Are you a real Christian—a follower of the Lamb? Have you been born again? Are you taking up your cross daily, denying yourself, and following after Him? Is your life counting for God and souls? Even when the wires of heavenly connection are up, you should inspect them carefully before coming for healing. It takes only a little bit of paper in the electric light socket to keep the light from shining. It only takes a little doubt, hardness, backbiting, criticism, unforgiveness, disobedience, or a grudge to hinder the blessed power of God from flowing into that life of yours. It is a very sacred thing to ask the divine touch of Jesus upon these mortal bodies of ours. There is no question as to the power being in the storehouse or as to our electric lightbulb needing the power; but, oh, make sure of the connection!

"Yes, yes," I hear someone cry, "I see that I have a real part to fill if I would receive my healing, but it has been so many years since I went to church or have taken any real interest in religion; just what must I do to be healed?"

Brother, Sister, dear, I trust that the first step you will take will be to fall so in love with Jesus the crucified that the healing of your body will be a secondary consideration. Seek first the kingdom of God and His righteousness, and all these things will be added unto you. (See Matthew 6:33.) Come to the altar, get down on your knees today, repent of your sins, turn to the Lord, and seek salvation.

"Oh, Sister, not at that altar!" someone exclaims. "Not here, where I am so well-known! People will talk about it so. I can pray better in my own room by my own bedside, I am quite sure."

Why, that is just what Naaman said: "*Are not Abana and Pharpar, rivers of Damascus, better than all the waters of Israel? May I not wash in them, and be clean?*" (2 Kings 5:12). Yet none other than those lowly, humble, despised waters brought healing to the leper. You have tried your own way and gotten but deeper into sorrow; why not come God's way—the way of the humble and lowly Nazarene who hung on the cross for you? Repent of your sins with a godly sorrow for sin. Do not glaze over the surface but go to the depths.

"Seek My face," calls the Savior. Oh, let your heart answer, "Your face, O Lord, will I seek." (See Psalm 27:8.) Hear the Master sweetly say, "Draw near unto Me, and I will draw near unto you." (See James 4:8.)

Why, He is running to meet you already with wide-open arms. "Poor, weary, sin-sick child," He is saying, "you have been wandering such a long, long time. You have been torn by the thorns and bruised by the jagged rocks. None other has been able to fill the hungry longing of your heart. Come closer to Me, child. Turn your back upon the world, with its bitterness and sin. Come closer to My wounded side and lay your head upon My breast. I will pardon your backsliding. I will forgive you freely. A clean heart will I give you, and a new spirit will I create within you. Your sins will I cast into the sea of My forgetfulness and remember them against you nevermore. Your cup will I fill to overflowing with the joy of salvation, and your head will I anoint with the oil of gladness. Seek My face, dear child! Let Me be your all and in all."

Glory to Jesus! When you get there, dear heart, the healing of your body will be but a secondary thought.

> Since mine eyes were fixed on Jesus,
> I've lost sight of all beside
> So enchained my spirit's vision,
> Gazing at the crucified.[2]

2. Mary D. James, "All for Jesus," 1871.

It is not money, nor arrogance, nor even hope that makes them clean and white, but implicit faith, humility, and obedience to the voice of the Lord.

The railroad track must be laid—every tie in place, every rail fastened, and the last spike driven, before the great transcontinental express can go through. It takes a great deal longer to lay the track than for the express to pass by.

In coming for healing, make sure of the condition of the track. You are inviting the express of God's unlimited power to come over. Remember that, in making railroads, the hills must be laid low and the valleys exalted; pride must flow down before Him, and the rough places must be made smooth. Do not spend so much time worrying and scolding because the train does not come more quickly. *You* care for the track—*God* will take care of the train.

Take the electric light, for instance. It is not enough to have an electric lightbulb in your possession—the wires must be strung and the connections properly made clear back to the powerhouse before the light can shine in your home.

Just so, it is not enough for you to say, "I have a body that needs healing, and I know that the Lord has the power to make me whole." That is like saying, "I have an electric lightbulb in my hand, and I know there is enough current in the powerhouse to make it a shining light, but what about the wires and connections between?"

Selfish motives are gone, and you are now drawing nearer every moment to the Great Physician who has power to heal the sick. The all-absorbing love for your newfound Christ and the overwhelming desire to be pleasing in His sight and to win jewels for His crown have taken the place of selfishness.

"And does this hinder one from seeking physical healing," you ask, "seeing that our eyes have been taken off our own suffering and fixed upon Christ?"

Ah, no! It will help you a thousand miles along the way. For, instead of asking healing for a selfish motive only, one now seeks life and strength, that one may the more fully and gladly serve and win other souls for this adorable Christ of Calvary.

The conflict is over, the battle ended. There is a *nevertheless not my will but Thine be done* in the soul. (See Luke 22:42.) "Dear Jesus, if You want me to go to heaven, I thank You that I know it is well with my soul. But if, oh Lord, it is Your will to spare me on this earth, I pray that I may have the strength and health, the power and wisdom, to win my family and others for You, dear Savior, and to be a shining light to those who sit in darkness."

If it is His good will to take one of the children home—amen! If not, bless the Lord, you can touch the hem of the Master's robe and have healing and strength for His service today, even as did they who lived when Jesus walked this earth. But whatsoever you do, whether you eat or drink, seek healing and strength, be sure that you do all for the glory of God. (See 1 Corinthians 10:31.) You can then look up as you come to the altar and, lifting your hands toward heaven, say:

> My body, soul and spirit
> Jesus, I give to Thee,
> A consecrated offering,
> Thine evermore to be.
> My all is on the altar,
> I'm waiting for the fire;
> Waiting, waiting, waiting,
> I'm waiting for the fire.[3]

Then remember, if you bring your gift to the altar and there remember that your brother has something against you, leave your gift before the altar and go first to be reconciled to your brother. Then come and offer your gift. (See Matthew 5:23–24.)

And when you stand praying, forgive—make those old-time grudges right. Go make it right with that one to whom you have not spoken for so long. Ask your wife to forgive the harsh words that have so often made the tears spring into her eyes. Forgive that enemy the injury you could never forgive before. (See Mark 11:25.) Otherwise, how can you pray, "Forgive us our trespasses, as we forgive those who trespass against us"? (See Matthew 6:12.)

"But what has all this to do with my receiving healing?" you ask. "I thought that all I had to do was to walk right up on that platform, be prayed for, and be healed without further obligation on my part. What has all this to do with it, anyway?"

---

3. Mary D. James, "Consecration," 1869.

Why don't you see, this is the stringing of the electric light wires between the bulb and the power house and the making sure of the proper connections. This is the laying of the track across the desert wastes or the tunneling through the mountains and making straight paths for His feet so that the mighty express of God's glory and power may pass through.

Seek *first* the kingdom of God and His righteousness, and all else will be added unto you. Put first things first. Spend time in prayer. Read your Bible carefully and prayerfully, especially Matthew, Mark, Luke, John, and the Acts of the Apostles, with reference to those whom Jesus healed, and see what part they had in obeying His command and in having active faith.

Establish family worship in your home. Do not wait till you are here but begin to serve Jesus even now, till joy and peace are flooding your heart. Faith is rising mountain high, and you have *prayed through* and gotten the witness; every wire is in place between the bulb and the powerhouse, and you are ready for the hand of prayer to turn the switch and let the current of God's power flow through.

Jesus

The next and greatest one concerned in your healing is, of course, the one to whom you are coming for healing—Jesus. Has He the power to heal? Is He willing to do so, and will He do His part?

Yes; beyond a doubt, He has the same power today as He had in the old days. His promises are constant. Amen to everyone who believes. When the leper in the Bible days said, "*If thou wilt, thou canst make me clean*" (Mark 1:40), and his healing depended upon the "willingness of Jesus," the Master, without hesitation, said, "*I will; be thou made clean*" (Mark 1:41). There is no doubt as to His *willingness*, if we only have the faith and ask for His glory.

As for Jesus *doing His part*, Brother, Sister, it was already done when He purchased our healing at the cruel whipping post almost nineteen hundred years ago, that, by His stripes, we might be healed (see 1 Peter 2:24), for "*himself took our infirmities, and bare our sicknesses*" (Matthew 8:17).

Just as in salvation, Christ has done *His* part in the finished work of Calvary and now awaits our coming to the cross in faith to accept and make this great redemption ours, so with divine healing, the Great Physician, the Son of Righteousness with healing in His wings, has done His part. He bore the cruel lash, carried our pain and suffering, was smitten of God and afflicted as our burden-bearer, and bore not only our sins but that dire result of sin—sickness and pain. Thus, with Isaiah, we can cry exultingly, *"He was wounded for our transgressions…and with his stripes we are healed"* (Isaiah 53:5).

Indeed, He will do His part. Draw near to Him, and He will draw near to you. (See James 4:8.) Reach out your hands in faith and touch the blessed hem of His garment, and He will bend low over you. You will feel the gentle pressure of His nail-pierced hand laid in healing and benediction upon your head. Jesus is the same yesterday, today and forever; He who heard the cry of His people in times past is just the same today. His ear has not grown heavy, that He cannot hear, nor has His arm been shortened, that it cannot save. (See Isaiah 59:1.)

The One Who Prays for You

The third party concerned in your healing is the one who anoints you with oil, according to James 5:14, and prays with you, that you might be made whole. Just what part is played by this one who prays for the sick, and of what importance is His role?

The first duty of the one who is instrumental in praying for the sick is the duty that Christ laid upon His disciples in John 10:49—namely, that of bringing the man near to Him. The blind man cried, *"Thou son of David, have mercy on me"* (Mark 10:47). He had faith. He had prayed through and reached the ear of the Master.

He had done his part.

Jesus was ready to do His part.

But a blessed duty, or part, in the healing was granted to the disciples when Jesus commanded them to bring the man near to Him. First, then, lift up Jesus from the earth. Talk of His power; magnify His name. Many take so much time talking about what Jesus *cannot* do that they spend very little time telling of the things He *can* do.

Sow the seed of faith in the hearts of the people, and have faith *yourself*. Those who pray for the healing of the sick should themselves first be partakers of the fruit and be a living example of what they preach, having a sound, whole body, and being invigorated by the strength and resurrection of the life of Jesus.

Bring the sufferer near to Christ in prayer, faith, and praise. Make Jesus so real through the preached Word that your audience can see His blessed face through the parting clouds and reach out their hands to touch Him.

Second, it is the sacred duty of those who pray for the sick to believe with the whole heart and have the real touch of God upon them, the Holy Spirit dwelling within them, and the authority of the Master clothing them as the raiment of Elijah clothed Elisha.

> *Let him ask in faith, nothing wavering, for he that wavereth is like a wave of the sea, driven with the wind and tossed. For let not that man think that he shall receive any thing of the Lord. A double minded man is unstable in all his ways.* (James 1:6–8)

One can tell in a moment whether a preacher, or the one who is exhorting or praying, has faith. Have you ever heard a man preach a long sermon and then say, "Now, *if* there is one here tonight who wants salvation, will you lift your hand and say, 'Pray for me'?"

Why, right there, his faith has wavered; he seldom gets more than the one he asked for, whereas the man of faith has won the day and cries, "Let *every* sinner or backslider in this building lift up your hand high, and by that lifted hand, say, 'Pray for me; *I* am a sinner and want salvation.' You all need Jesus! Let everyone lift his hands and say so." Have you watched the hands go up? And have you seen the hundreds of penitents weeping their way to the altars? So it is in the prayer for the sick. According to your faith, so will it be done to you.

In a recent meeting, we came to the closing day, and thousands were still waiting to be prayed for, so it became necessary for various groups, composed of some twenty ministers, to be called upon to offer prayer for the healing of the afflicted. Among the long lines of sufferers came a deaf man, desiring prayer that his hearing might be restored. A certain dear minister, who perhaps had never before been called upon to pray for deaf ears to be unstopped, began to talk to the Lord about His power and willingness to hear the prayers of His people. After a few moments, he looked at the man and, realizing that something definite should be done, leaned over inquiringly, brought his lips close to the ear in question, and asked, "O deaf ear, are you going to open? Are you?" Right there, he had wavered, and let not that man who wavers think that he will obtain anything from God! With the unction and power of the Holy Spirit upon him, he should have commanded, "O deaf ear, in the name of the Lord Jesus Christ, I *command* you to be opened and to hear the Word of the Lord! You deaf spirit, come out of him, in the mighty name of Jesus." Ask in faith, nothing wavering, and it will be done *according to your faith.*

Tell the one for whom you pray to have faith also, reaching out and clasping the promise to hold it tightly, and it will be his. Whether he is healed instantly or gradually, he must believe from that very hour.

Third, the one who prays for the sick should have clean hands and a pure heart.

Many ministers we know are using tobacco. Throw it away; let your own heart be cleansed with the precious blood and your lips be sweet and pure before you pray reverently the prayer of faith. Could you imagine Jesus smoking a big cigar and then going in to pray for the afflicted?

Do not expect to spend your time telling or listening to foolish, idle stories or gossip, or being a good mixer in the club, and then rushing into His presence to bring the power down. Keep close to Jesus yourself. Keep the lamp of faith brightly burning. Walk with God like Enoch of old, till your life is swallowed up in His own blessed will. Let triumphant faith mount up and up till your own face is all aglow, and poor, weak, tempest-driven souls see in you that mighty, unwavering confidence and trust in God that will give new courage and guide them into the calm, safe harbor of the Savior's strength and blessing.

Do not feel, however, dear, afflicted soul, that unless the preacher or elder who prays does his part, that you need necessarily go away without healing. Many are healed in answer to their own prayers while seated in the audience or while praying in their homes. *"Is any among you afflicted? let him pray"* (James 5:13). Even though you are alone, you can reach up right where you are and claim the promise. It is only natural, however, and perfectly scriptural, to want someone to pray the prayer of faith for you and to hold up your hands in encouragement as you come to God, for we also read:

> *Is any sick among you? let him call for the elders of the church; and let them pray over him, anointing him with oil in the name of the Lord: and the prayer of faith shall save the sick, and the Lord shall raise him up, and if he have committed sins, they shall be forgiven him.* (James 5:14–15)

Let us, therefore, do our part. Press in close to the Master—the Great Physician—the Shepherd of the sheep, who stands waiting with his flask of oil to make us whole in body, soul, and spirit. There is not a tear so blinding, but Jesus can wipe it away. There is not a hurt so deep in the heart, but He can comfort and bless. There is not a body so weary, so weak, and so sick, but His touch can strengthen and heal. There is not a load so heavy or a burden so great, but His love can lift and bear it away.

5

HOW TO RECEIVE
YOUR HEALING

T*hy faith hath made thee whole"* (Matthew 9:22). *"According to your faith be it done unto you"* (Matthew 9:29). *"Woman, great is thy faith: be it unto thee even as thou wilt"* (Matthew 15:28). These were the words of the Master when He trod the shores of Galilee.

It was faith that made the believer whole in Bible days, and it is faith to reach up and touch the hem of the Master's seamless dress that can make us whole today. For *"if ye have faith as a grain of mustard seed,"* said Jesus, *"ye shall say unto this mountain, Remove hence to yonder place, and it shall remove; and nothing shall be impossible unto you"* (Matthew 17:20).

In order to get this living, active, mountain-moving faith in Jesus Christ, you must get on believing ground. Faith comes by hearing the Word of God. (See Romans 10:17.) To rightfully understand and feed upon the Word, the heart must be given to the Lord Jesus. We must be washed in the precious blood, be born again, and be no longer children of darkness but children of light.

"Well, if the Lord heals me, I'll believe and be converted," we hear someone say.

But, dear one, this is not the attitude in which to come to the Great Physician, Jesus. He did not heal the sick under those conditions when He was on earth. Healing was not received first and faith afterward, but faith first and then healing, for He said, *"Thy faith hath made thee whole"* (Matthew 9:22). But to a sinful nation who seeks a sign, no sign will be given. (See Matthew 12:39.) Neither can one bargain with the Lord and exchange service for healing. Many forget their vows and promises to God after the answer has come.

Be Born Again

Positively, the first thing to do is to be genuinely born again—not for the sake of being healed but because of real heart conviction for sin and the wooing, all-conquering love of Jesus Christ.

Many have been not a little surprised and filled with questions when, in our meetings, we have listed a complete surrender to Jesus—a change of heart and a bright salvation experience—as one of the conditions required for us to pray for the healing of the sick and afflicted. But, you see, it is Jesus and not us whom the afflicted must look to for healing. It is to Him that they must pray.

Think for a moment—how *could* a sinner pray to the Lord for healing? If he were really honest, he would have to pray something like this:

Oh, Lord Jesus, I am a sinner. I know You have long been knocking at my heart's door and that I have never been willing to let You in. Even now, I am unwilling to deny myself or to take up my cross and follow You, but while I am not ready to live for You or to repent of the coldness and sin that grieves Your heart—and though I am rejecting You and unwilling to do anything for You—I would like You, please dear Lord, to do something for me. Please heal my broken body so that I may go out to better enjoy the world. Heal my eyes so that I can the better see the moving pictures. Open my deaf ears so that I may enjoy the devil's jokes and gossip. Heal my crippled hands so that I can play cards or work for my own selfish ends, and heal my feet so that I might dance and run in worldly paths!

Oh, no, those might not be the exact words uttered by the petitioning sinner's lips, but it would be the language of the heart, would it not? And, after all, it is upon the heart that the Lord looks, and it does not seem possible that the Lord *could* answer that prayer for the honor and glory of His own dear name, does it?

Make an Out-and-out Surrender

Give Him your heart, freely and gladly. Drink deep from the joyous wells of His salvation till your heart overflows with the rich fullness of His love. Then, come crying:

Dear Jesus, my Savior and my Lord, Your name do I worship and adore. By Your blood I have been redeemed. My whole heart and life flows out to You in gladness and surrender for service great or small. Take me and use me, I pray. But, oh, dear Lord, this body is sick and frail. I come to You for healing and strength, that I may serve You better and help lead souls from darkness into light. Heal my eyes, that I may read the blessed Book; my ears, that I may hear the preached Word; my hands, that I may minister in loving deeds to those in need; my feet, that they may run to do Your bidding, Savior dear. Humbly, I ask in faith for Your own glory. Dear Lord, I *do* believe and take Your promise *now*.

There is quite a difference in the heart language of those two prayers, is there not? And it does seem as though one could pray this latter prayer with much more assurance and confidence.

Do not seek salvation for the sake of being healed; but after seeking and finding the Savior, then come for deliverance from sickness and pain that you may henceforth live for Him who died for you.

Having read of the miracles of healing our Lord has performed, people often rush into the meetings from distant places, saying, "Pray for me quick,

Sister; I have to catch a train or leave for home tomorrow." But they have not sat long under the preaching of the gospel till, when asked if they feel that they are now ready to go to the altar for prayer, they almost invariably reply, "Oh, no, let me wait a day longer. I have a few more letters to write asking forgiveness, a few more things to make right, a couple of more bills to pay, and so forth." Bless the Lord, the Spirit has been working in their hearts, and instead of rushing pell-mell without thought or preparation into the most holy and righteous presence of the King of Kings, asking His pure, nail-pierced hands to be laid upon their sinful, selfish bodies, they are coming now with clean hands and a pure heart, entering humbly under the covering of the precious blood.

Do Not Come on Your Own Merits

"But I have been such a wicked sinner," some other heart may cry. "My life has been wasted. Would He ever hear my cry? Would He save, heal, and baptize me with His precious Holy Spirit? Am I not too sinful, sick, and broken of body and soul?"

Indeed, He will hear your cry, dear one. He came not to call the righteous but sinners to repentance. You are just the one whom He will hear. When Jesus walked this earth, none was too sinful for Him to save, none too sick for Him to heal.

And it has been a noticeable fact that the new convert, filled with humility and a sense of his own unworthiness, often receives healing much more quickly than those who have been Christian workers for many years and who now come of their own merits, filled with a sense of their own goodness and importance.

"Why, I am Mr. So-and-so. I've done this, that, and the other for the Lord for so many years, and I am sure that He will heal me." But oh, it is not upon our own merits, righteousness, or even service that we can claim the promise; for all that we have done, after all, is but our reasonable service. It is the merits and righteousness of Jesus that we must plead. Coming in humility, we find that, indeed, when we are weak, then are we strong, for He resists the proud but gives grace to the humble. (See 1 Corinthians 4:10; James 4:6.)

"Have you faith that Jesus will heal you now?" we often ask the sick who come for prayer. When dealing with old Christians, we frequently meet the following complacent, self-satisfied answer in a tone that would indicate that they almost resented the fact that we felt the necessity of such a question:

"Oh my, yes! Why, I have always had faith."

"How long have you been ill, Sister, and crippled up in this wheelchair?"

"About ten years."

"And yet you say, in an offhand, assured way, with a little wave of your hand, 'Oh yes, indeed, I have always had faith.' Why don't you see, my dear, that if you really had faith—that is, the instantaneous, mountain-moving faith for the fraction of a second—the work would be *done*, and this captive body would be free? Get out of that self-satisfied, boastful complacency and—in humility, heart searching, and earnest prayer—draw near with sincerity and unfeigned faith unto the Lord."

The Difference Between Passive Faith and Active Faith

Having been converted, having made peace with the brother who had something against you, as far as it is in your power, and having put your all upon the altar in sacrifice, you are now coming to Christ for healing.

Come with radiant, active faith; pray earnestly; pray believing, doubting nothing, and you will feel the mighty hand upon your life. His power will thrill through your being, and the same Spirit that raised Jesus from the dead will quicken your mortal body. (See Romans 8:11.)

"Just what do you mean by 'active' faith? Is there more than one kind of faith?" I hear someone ask.

Yes; there is passive faith, and there is active faith. There is an instantaneous faith that takes the promise now. There is a steady, unwavering faith that can stand the test and, though the vision tarry, wait for it, growing daily in strength as young trees grow in stature. The one with passive faith says, "I will be prayed for, and *if* it is His will to heal me, I will be restored to health"—but right there is an *if*, small in itself, but a most mighty stumbling block to faith.

Had the woman with the issue of blood sat by the wayside, saying, "Well, if it is His will to heal me, I am willing. I will just sit here at ease, and if He happens to come to me and heal me, all right; if not, all right, but I will make no great effort until He does," do you think she would ever have been made whole? It was her active faith that *pressed through* the throng and touched the Master's robe that brought about her healing.

Passive faith just stands there and lets someone else do all the praying, *hoping* to be healed and willing for it, if it comes, but making no real effort to reach out and take it by active faith. *Hope*, however, is *not faith*, though many mistake the one for the other.

An Example of the Difference Between the Two

Let me tell you the true story of something that happened in one of our meetings that exemplifies the difference between active and passive faith.

During the great revival campaign in the Memorial Hall of Dayton, Ohio, the Lord graciously poured His Spirit upon us in a most marvelous way. Thousands were seeking the Lord as their Savior, Healer, and Baptizer.

The auditorium was packed almost to suffocation. The basement also was filled. Policemen and firemen were struggling with the multitudes that thronged the streets outside. Healthy friends who carried the sick and had been crowded out had, in desperation resorted to cutting out the basement windows and passing in their afflicted on beds to those within. From early morning until late at night, the throngs continued to stand. And now, within the building, on the great platform, prayer was still being offered for the sick.

Many mighty healings were resulting. Deaf ears were unstopped, and the lame had been made to leap for joy. As quickly as one row of supplicants was prayed for, another would take its place. We who were praying for the sick turned now to the new row.

The first was a man with a stout walking stick in his hand, whose limb was held painfully and straight before him. The man appeared to have absolutely no burden of prayer but was sitting up straight in his chair, gazing about him with wide open eyes, watching the workers and the people as they came and went. I looked at him searchingly with the thought that is ever uppermost in the mind when praying for the sick: *Has he faith—active, mountain-moving faith?* I was afraid that he did not.

Second in the line was a dear lady with a child perhaps three or four years of age seated upon her lap. One arm was pressed tightly about the child; the other was raised to heaven. Her lips moved in audible prayer, and tears flowed down her cheeks. Her face—there was no doubt as to faith there!

The Man with the Cane

Addressing first the elderly man with the inexpressive face and the open eyes, I asked, "Well, Brother, dear, have you faith that Jesus will heal you now?"

"Why, I certainly *hope* He will," he made answer.

"But, Brother, have you only a 'hope so' faith? No assurance from the Lord?"

"Why, why, I thought perhaps I could be healed; I certainly hope so."

"Just what is your greatest reason for desiring healing, Brother?" I asked, trying another track.

"Why, to be rid of the pain, of course," he answered testily.

"But isn't it even just a little bit so that you could serve the Lord and work for Him with all your heart and strength?" I persisted.

"W-e-e-ll, I suppose so." He spoke hesitatingly, without conviction, as though the thought were foreign. The man had a hard, selfish face, and we could not help wondering whether he had ever made a real sacrifice for the Lord Jesus in his life.

There was nothing to do but to offer a prayer for the man, of course. But, oh, that living, vital faith one so covets when praying for the afflicted seemed to have been sinking away down out of sight, and all we could do, after we had prayed, was to turn to the man and say, "According to your faith be it done unto you."

"Now, Brother," we tried to smile bright encouragement, "do you take the promise? Come! Rise to your feet, in Jesus' name. If you but have faith, you can walk from this platform straight and strong and every bit whole, leaving your cane behind you."

As I spoke, I succeeded in getting him to his feet; faith was springing up in my own heart, and I had the assurance that, even now, if he could but grasp the promise, he would be made whole.

"Come, Brother! Forget the cane, lean upon the Lord, and walk, in Jesus' name!"

"Oh-h-h! But I *couldn't* walk without the cane, Sister! My limb has been sore so long," he cried in a startled voice, without even trying to walk, and taking a tighter grasp upon his cane.

We groaned within our spirits, and the man, clinging to the stick, hobbled away. Only a moment, however, could be spared in following him with a regretful gaze. Hundreds of others were waiting for prayer—hundreds who would have real, active faith.

The Mother and the Paralyzed Child

Next in line was the mother with the little daughter who had been afflicted with infantile paralysis.

The mother's lips were still moving in prayer, as, with closed eyes and tear-stained cheeks, she clasped her child to her breast and rocked gently to and fro with an intensity of emotion and faith that appeared to be oblivious to all surroundings. I scarcely needed to ask the question here, "Mother, dear, have you faith that Jesus will heal the little darling now and make her walk and run again?"

She opened eyes that were red with weeping but in which glowed a light kindled by the taper of faith, and she cried, "Indeed, I have faith, Sister. I have *prayed through*. I just *know* that it will be done. This paralysis must go. My child will walk, in Jesus' name."

Ah, what blessed faith had she! Jesus spoke of those like her, saying, "I have not seen such faith; no, not in all Israel." With every word she uttered, we could feel our own faith mounting. No long prayer needed here! The praying had been done in advance.

"According to your faith be it done unto you. In the name of the Lord Jesus Christ, be made whole!"

"Put the little darling down on her feet, Mother dear. Dry your tears and take your little girl by the hand. She will walk." And she did, too. Only Mama went too slow, and the pretty little darling let go the mother's hand and ran and danced across the platform, perfectly whole. What a novelty it was to have that paralyzed side paralyzed no longer! How grand to use that little foot! She would run a little, then stop short, lift up the foot, look at it inquiringly and approvingly, then skip some more, like a little lamb gamboling in the field, then stop again and turn the foot in all directions, gazing at it delightedly, before she ran and danced some more. The delighted audience laughed and shouted and wept all in the same breath.

The happy mother lifted up her clasped hands and cried, "Oh, Jesus! I just knew You'd do it! I just *knew* it! And oh, I thank You, Lord. I will give You my love, my strength, my all, and ever bring her up in Your paths, dear Savior."

Do you see the difference, dear one? Here was a woman with active faith. She cried, and the Lord heard her; and according to her faith, she received.

Don't Lose Faith if Healing Is Not Instantaneous

Very often the Lord heals His children instantaneously, and yet there are some who are healed gradually and begin to mend from that hour. In these cases, active faith is more necessary than ever.

This was exemplified by our dear Sister Fraga, of Dayton, Ohio, whom so many have learned to know and love. She came to the meeting on crutches. She was frightfully deformed, with dislocated hips, which had been out of their sockets for years. When prayed for, she reached out to Jesus in simple, childlike faith and said that she could feel the hips snapping back into place. She let the crutches fall from under her arms and, declaring that she was healed, walked away, something she had not been able to do before.

But, though the hips were gradually going back into the sockets, the body was still far from straight, and we used to catch our breath when Mrs. Fraga rose to testify (as she tended to do at each testimony meeting) and declare that she was healed. Then, gradually, day by day, as this precious sister turned her house into a home of prayer, brought her husband to Jesus, prayed with sinners at the altar, and went out for miles to pray for and bring others to the meetings, her lameness began to disappear.

We saw this dear sister one year after she had been prayed for, and she was as trim and as straight as a girl. She was still ministering to the sick and afflicted, walking for miles with perfect ease, for, as she said, "Only those who have been in trouble, bound with braces of steel and leather, tortured by crutches and pain, could ever fully sympathize and yearn with such a full heart to help those who walk in the path of affliction."

Here again was active faith that stepped out on the promise, even as Peter stepped out on the water and walked to meet the Lord. This woman had held fast through sunshine and tempest, believing that He who had begun the good work was also able to perfect it. (See Philippians 1:6.)

Have Faith in God

Remember that faith is not always accompanied by feeling. Faith is the substance of things hoped for, the evidence of things not seen. (See Hebrews 11:1.) Whether you are healed instantly or gradually, hold fast to the promise. In the Bible we read of some who came to Jesus and were healed as they went. (See, for example, Luke 17:12–14.) Just so today, there are some who see little visible indication of healing at the moment they are prayed for. But this is the very time to have faith and to hold fast. If they should wait a moment or so, without feeling any great surge of healing power, and then walk away with downcast face, saying, "Oh, I was prayed for a moment ago, but I *feel* no different; I guess this is not for me," then, according to their faith will it be done. Remember, *faith is not feeling*, and trust is not trace. Keep your eyes on Jesus, who is at this very moment measuring and testing the quantity and quality of your faith.

Cling to the words of Isaiah: *"With his stripes we are healed"* (Isaiah 53:5). Lift your heart to Jesus and say, "By Your own suffering at the whipping post, You bore my sickness and pain. My eyes are upon You, dear Lord. By faith I lay hold of the promise. The work is completed in You. Complete it now in me, O Lord."

Step Out Boldly upon the Promise

Pray through before you come to Christ for healing. Then come with perfect faith in Jesus and His power to heal. When you lay aside that cane or those crutches, after prayer, do not put one foot out hesitatingly and say, "Um, now, I wonder, could I take a step on that foot? I wonder if I could I bear my weight on it? It's been a pretty sore foot! Now, let's see…I'm going to try."

No! No! That is not faith!

Do you suppose that Peter would ever have been able to walk on the water to meet his Lord if he had put one foot rather dubiously on the wave and said, "Let's see now…I wonder if that water will bear my weight? I know that the Lord bade me come, but this water is pretty soft, and I'm pretty heavy, but I'll try it and see"?

Why, no; he would have sunk in a moment! It was faith that kept Peter up—faith in Jesus. As soon as he got his eyes off the Christ and fixed them fearfully upon the tempestuous waves, or the circumstances with which he was surrounded, he began to sink.

According to your faith, it will be done to you. Do not fix your eyes upon your own condition or surroundings. Fix your eyes on Jesus. Have faith and walk to meet Him in gladsome love and service, and the answer will come.

Going Home to Heaven

"But suppose that it is not His will to heal me? Suppose He wants to take me home to heaven?"

Well, amen! That is a different matter. Your coronation day is at hand. Blessed are those who die in the Lord.

Paul was in a strait as to whether it was better to stay in order to serve and minister unto his brethren or to depart, declaring that to be absent from the body is to be present with the Lord. (See 2 Corinthians 5:6–8.) If the Savior has spoken to your heart and is calling you home, hallelujah, there is nothing to fear, if your heart is washed in the blood of the Lamb. For you, death has lost its sting, and the grave its victory. (See 1 Corinthians 15:55.) When you pass through the waters, the Lord will be with you, and the waters will not overflow. (See Isaiah 43:2.)

But we do believe that the Lord's little children do not need to die screaming with convulsions and pain. We read of our fathers that they "fell asleep." (See, for example, Acts 13:36.)

> Safe in the arms of Jesus,
> Safe on His gentle breast;
> There by His love protected,
> Sweetly my soul shall rest.[4]

If you have the blessed assurance that the Lord is calling you to that golden shore, you will, of course, be longing and ready to go; but if, on the other hand, you still have years to spend below, there is work to be done. Thousands on every hand are perishing in sin. You can be quickened and healed and made every bit whole through Jesus' mighty power, and you can then go forth into service, great or small, be it at home or abroad. You may become a soulwinner for the Master, that when He calls you, you will not be empty-handed.

In gazing upon the sinner who has just given his heart to Jesus and, in his illness, is very near the other shore, this verse always comes to my mind:

> Must I go, and empty-handed,
> Thus my dear Redeemer meet?
> Bring no soul with which to greet Him,
> Lay no trophies at His feet?[5]

---

4. Fanny Crosby, "Safe in the Arms of Jesus," 1868.
5. Charles C. Luther, "Must I Go, and Empty Handed," 1877.

How I covet at least a few months of service for those who, when the last summons comes, will "come rejoicing, bringing in the sheaves."[6] (See Psalm 126:6.)

Oh, the multitudes we have seen come to Jesus for healing! Our ears still ring with the glad shout of the blind when they received their sight and cried aloud, "Oh, I can see! I can see. Dear people, dear Jesus, I can see again." We still see the overjoyed, almost rapt, expression of those whose deaf ears were suddenly opened, so that they were liberated from a tomb of silence and enabled to hear the songs of praise to Jesus and the voices of their loved ones. Again we can see the lame, leaping and fairly dancing for joy, their crutches, braces, and canes being thrown away. Hear the testimonies of those whose cancers and tumors have melted away.

Step into Bethesda's pool by faith today, dear heart, and your faith will make you whole.

6. Knowles Shaw, "Bringing in the Sheaves," 1874.

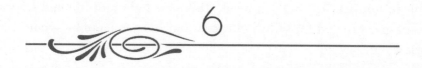

6

HOW TO KEEP YOUR HEALING

Having received your healing from the loving hand of Jesus, the next thing is to *keep it.*

"Oh! Is there a possibility of losing my healing after receiving it?" you ask.

"Is there a possibility of a discharged patient, who has just recovered from pneumonia, going out into the blasts of wintry winds and coming down with double pneumonia, so that his latter condition is worse than the former?

"Is there a possibility of a sinner coming to this altar for conversion, being washed in the blood of Jesus and forgiven of his sin, going out into the world among godless companions, and forgetting his vows to the Lord?"

"Why, yes; we hear of such things every day."

"Then it is also possible for people to receive the divine healing touch of Jesus Christ upon their bodies and then to depart from His paths into doubt, criticism, and sin, eventually not only losing the healing but even becoming more ill than before."

Remember that Christ is the Vine, and we are the branches. In healing, as in salvation, we have no separate life of our own. In Him we move and live and have our being. (See Acts 17:28.) Sever the branch from the Vine, and it is bound to perish and wither away.

Jesus said: *"Behold, thou art made whole: sin no more, lest a worse thing come unto thee"* (John 5:14).

The very hour in which your healing has begun, look about you and begin to minister to those in need. This new light and life and strength are not given to you for selfish purposes but to spend and be spent in His service.

When Jesus touched the hand of Peter's mother-in-law, the fever left her, and *"she arose, and **ministered** unto them"* (Matthew 8:15.) Will you not do the same? For every bit of strength you give Him, He will repay you a hundred-fold. Hallelujah!

Walk in the Holy Spirit; spend much time in reading His Word and seeking His face in prayer, but no time in doubtful disputations.

Give not only of your love and service but of your *means* to Jesus, also. A man came into one of the meetings one time on crutches. He was on his way to San Francisco, where he was to undergo a surgical operation upon his limb. The Lord graciously healed him in answer to prayer. The man was overjoyed as he hung his crutches upon a nearby post in the tabernacle. His joy, however, was not only in the fact that the painful operation was no longer necessary but also that he had saved five hundred dollars. But oh, could he have poured those five hundred dollars into the treasuries of the Lord for foreign missionary work or the spreading of the gospel at home, how much more blessed a thank offering that would have been. In fact, this would have been but his *"reasonable service"* (Romans 12:1). Anything he gave above this would have been a thank offering. Give, and it will be given unto you, a good measure, heaped up and running over. (See Luke 6:38.)

Establish a family altar in your home, and keep the light brightly burning. Begin today to win others for Christ. Do not try to see how *little* but how *much* you can do and give.

It is, I repeat, a very sacred thing to ask the divine touch of the Lord upon these mortal bodies, and if we want keep our physical healing, we should walk with the Master.

Through correspondence and through *The Bridal Call*[7], we have been enabled to keep in personal touch with large numbers of those converted and healed in the meetings. A great cloud of witnesses are standing true after several years have elapsed and are still permanently healed.

On the other hand, there are some who were mightily touched by God who have *lost* their healing. Such a one was a young man in Illinois, whose paralysis was healed instantaneously in answer to prayer in a meeting held in a Methodist church there.

Delightedly he slung his crutches over his shoulder and strode down the aisle, smiling broadly. From the meeting he went to the back room of a worldly place of amusement, in which his old companions in sin were playing a game of poker and gambling. After having shown them how easily he could walk without his crutches and having paced the room several times with ease, he sat down at their insistent urging, dealt the cards, procured his stack of chips, played the game, and gambled with them.

In the midst of the game, the numbness flowed back into his limbs, and the paralysis returned. He not only lost his healing but was worse than before.

Go your way and sin no more—lest a worse thing come upon you.

The Lord did not promise His blessing and protection to the sinner and the scornful but promised His blessing to…

> …*the man that walketh not in the counsel of the ungodly, nor standeth in the way of sinners, nor sitteth in the seat of the scornful. But his delight is in the law of the* Lord; *and in his law doth he meditate day and night.*
> (Psalm 1:1–2)

To him who walks closely with God and meditates on His law (that is, reads His Word, the Bible, and thinks upon it earnestly), He promises that he "*shall be like a tree planted by the rivers of water, that bringeth forth his fruit in his season; his leaf also shall not wither; and whatsoever he doeth shall prosper*" (Psalm 1:3).

But if, instead of walking a holy, sober, God-fearing life with Jesus, the man goes back to his theater, dance hall, card party, seat of the scornful, and

---

7. A monthly magazine produced by the author.

selfish life not lived for the glory of God, the branch is severed from the true Vine, and this protection and abounding life and strength are not promised to him, for *"the ungodly are not so: but are like the chaff which the wind driveth away…for the* LORD *knoweth the way of the righteous: but the way of the ungodly shall perish"* (Psalm 1:4, 6).

I would not dare come to the altar for anointing and prayer for healing unless solemnly from that hour I pledged heart and life to do His bidding and meant to walk in His blessed way.

Avoid foolish talk, idle conversation, gossip, and criticism. There is not a more deadly enemy to the health of soul and body than an ungoverned tongue. It is as though one had pumped water from the river into a great reservoir, for life and irrigation purposes, and then foolishly opened the gates of the sluice box and let it all run back into the river again.

It is possible to talk, jest, or criticize away, between meetings, all the strength, blessing, and healing one has gained in those meetings.

A society woman was one of the many to be healed in Denver, Colorado. Her deaf ears were instantly unstopped in answer to prayer, and she went away rejoicing.

Sometime later, however, she returned with all the joy and light gone and complained to my mother that the healing was not permanent and that the deafness had gradually returned after a few days.

Mother looked thoughtfully at the lady awhile, as she stood there, dressed in the height of fashion, and then questioned her as to how she had been occupying her time since being prayed for.

"Why, just doing the ordinary things," she replied in a surprised tone, as though wondering what that had to do with the subject.

"Such as what?" my mother questioned persistently.

"Just the duties entailed by my social standing."

"Bridge parties, I presume?"

"Oh, certainly!"

"Theaters, parties, a ball, a new fashionable evening dress, a little gossip and exchanging of idle nothings over the teacups?"

"Why, yes," she admitted. "Just the usual things—"

But right there, Mother had put her finger on the reason for the woman's losing her healing. It means something to *keep* your healing.

Pray, read your Bible, spend and be spent in His service, testify as to what He has done for you, and resist the enemy when he assails.

Testify

Testify at every possible opportunity as to what the Lord has done for you. "*They overcame him* [the enemy] *by the blood of the Lamb, and by the word of their testimony*" (Revelation 12:11), we are told of those triumphantly sweeping up the glory way. Exalt the power of the Lord Jesus. Give Him glory and praise for what He has done.

Remember the ten lepers whom Jesus cleansed. Only one came back to bear witness. The Lord said, "*Were there not ten cleansed? but where are the nine?*" (Luke 17:17). Will you be the one to return with the testimony? You will find indeed that with each note of victory that you sound forth, added strength will be given you.

Resist Temptation

Do not imagine for a moment that the devil will allow such a great victory as that which has been wrought in your life to be accomplished without resistance. Every inch of ground will be disputed. He has several methods of attack.

One of his methods is to raise unbelievers about you who will try to sow the seed of doubt in the heart, just at the time when you stand most in need of help and encouragement.

Another is to bring back the old symptoms and twinges of pain, saying, "Aha! You thought you were healed, didn't you? But look at these waves piling up on every side. You cannot walk upon these waters much longer. Don't you feel that pain? Doesn't that prove that you are not healed?"

But keep your eyes upon Jesus. Lift up your heart and begin to praise the Lord; resist the devil, and he will flee from you. (See James 4:7.) Do not let the enemy corner you in a doubting castle; keep out, in the sunshine of Jesus' smile. Lift your voice in audible praise to Jesus and prove indeed that the "*joy of the Lord is your strength*" (Nehemiah 8:10). Remember that all things are possible for those who believe and that faith is the master key that opens the door of every promise castle of God's Word.

Another ruse of the enemy is to take the eyes of the Lord's children off of the righteousness of Jesus and the finished work of Calvary and to fix them upon their own imperfections and blemishes.

A dear young lady was taken from a bed in which she had lay suffering for a year and a half, following seven abdominal operations. After consecrating her life to Jesus, this beautiful girl (at that time little more than skin and bones) was prayed for. Jesus healed her of intestinal disorders and adhesions. For months, she walked in victory, enjoying more liberty and real happiness than she had ever known, for she had been afflicted since childhood.

Then came the time when she was preparing to attend a big revival meeting, in the very city in which her victory had been gained, to give her testimony.

Could the enemy allow this without a struggle? No! He came in like a flood with recurring symptoms of old-time pain, and when the dear sister lifted troubled eyes and asked why this had come, the devil began to accuse her, declaring that she must have done something wrong, failed somewhere, or fallen into sin.

Ah, how cunning the enemy is! Full well he knows that if he can get our eyes off of the righteousness of Jesus and center them upon our own unworthiness, we will sink like Peter of old. Each time her tender conscience would cringe and say, "Oh! I must have sinned or have done *something* wrong, though I do not know what it can be," the lash would fall again on her quivering spirit and the clouds roll more thickly over her sky.

At last, she came to us about the subject, asking that we would pray and inquire of the Lord regarding where the trouble lay. She stated that she had searched her heart, read the Word, and cried out to the Lord, and that though she knew she must have sinned terribly in some way, somehow, she did not know where the trouble lay.

In prayer, the Lord showed me that the devil was still the accuser of the brethren today, as in the days of old. (See Revelation 12:10.) Gathering the trembling little form into my arms, I told her that it was the devil and not the Lord who stood over her with the stinging lash and the threatening, intimidating air, saying, "Now, you bad girl, you have sinned somewhere. You have prayed and wept and done the best you knew; but, though I will not show you what it is, you have done something wrong somewhere and must suffer for it."

"Oh, darling," I said, "does this sound like the voice of Jesus? No! His voice is loving and tender. When He speaks, He says, 'Come, poor, tired child, and lay your head upon My breast. Let Me enfold you with My love and wrap you about with My presence and support. Gaze upon meme; listen to my words till your soul is filled with music and you are transformed into My own image.'

"Here, you have been listening to the enemy all this time. Every time you spoke, you put your hand to your ear, bent closer to him, and said, 'What did you say, devil? What's that you say?'

"Oh, my dear, listen to him no more! Resist the oppression of the evil one. Throw his yoke from off your neck. He whom the Son sets free is free indeed! Rise up and take your liberty."

She saw the light through the clouds and rose up in victory. The pain was gone. The enemy fled like vanquished shades of night before the rising sun of the morning, and *she was free*. The enemy had come in like a flood, but the Lord had raised a standard against him. (See Isaiah 59:19.)

This young lady attended the revival and became an active winner of souls; by her testimony, she reached the hearts and ears of thousands.

Hold Fast to the Promise

Hold fast to the promise, seeking His glory. "*He will not suffer thy foot to be moved: he that keepeth thee will not slumber*" (Psalm 121:3). "*Thou wilt keep him in perfect peace, whose mind is stayed on thee*" (Isaiah 26:3). If you hold fast to Him, He will hold fast to you, for He has promised that…

Because thou hast kept the word of my patience, I also will keep thee from the hour of temptation, which shall come upon all the world, to try them that dwell upon the earth. (Revelation 3:10)

Now unto him that is able to keep you from falling, and to preserve you faultless before the presence of his glory with exceeding joy, the only wise God our Savior, be glory and majesty, dominion and power, both now and for ever. Amen. (Jude 24–25)

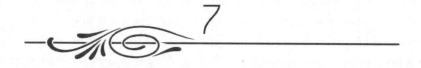

QUESTIONS FREQUENTLY ASKED REGARDING DIVINE HEALING

What Is Divine Healing?

It is the divine power of Jesus Christ to heal the sick and the afflicted in answer to the prayers of His people, without the aid of medicine or surgery, even as He did almost nineteen hundred years ago when He walked upon this earth.

Is Divine Healing for Today?

Many of God's dear children have the mistaken idea that the day of miracles is past and that the Lord Jesus no longer heals the sick. They have honestly believed, and some have even preached, that these things were only for Bible days, that Christ has now withdrawn this power (which, they say, was only given as a sign to the Jews), and that we now must do the best we can for these human bodies, looking for help from doctors, surgeons, medicines, herbs, massage, morphine, quacks—in fact, to anybody or anything except the Lord Jesus Christ, who is now either no longer willing or too far away to be troubled by such minor matters as the healing of the physical infirmities of His people.

But there is not one verse or passage in the dear old Bible to substantiate such a teaching. Not only were the sick healed in the Old Testament by looking to the Christ who was to come, and not only did Jesus heal the sick when He walked this earth, but He left explicit instructions with His disciples and followers that they, too, were to declare the good news of healing for the body as they preached the gospel: *"Into whatsoever city ye enter...heal the sick that are therein, and say unto them, The kingdom of God is come nigh unto you"* (Luke 10:8–9).

And he said unto them, Go ye into all the world, and preach the gospel to every creature. He that believeth and is baptized shall be saved; but he that believeth not shall be damned. And these signs shall follow them that believe; In my name shall they cast out devils; they shall speak with new tongues; They shall take up serpents; and if they drink any deadly thing, it shall not hurt them; they shall lay hands on the sick, and they shall recover. (Mark 16:15–18)

The disciples prayed for the healing of the sick throughout their entire ministries, and in closing, they left instructions for the church that, if there were any sick among them, they were to call for the elders of the church.

Let them pray over him, anointing him with oil in the name of the Lord. And the prayer of faith shall save the sick, and the Lord shall raise him up; and if he have committed sins, they shall be forgiven him. Confess your faults one to another, and pray for one another, that ye may be healed. The effectual fervent prayer of a righteous man availeth much. (James 5:14–16)

There are hundreds of promises about the continued power and unchangeableness of Jesus—who is the same yesterday, today, and forever (see Hebrews 3:18)—as to the abiding power of His Word and the assurance that no good gift is to be withheld from them that walk uprightly, but there is never a hint that His arm was to be shortened or his power no longer available for the healing of the sick after the passing away of the apostles.

Beyond a doubt, divine healing is for today. If we preach the same gospel of power that Peter preached in Acts 5, we can see the same signs and wonders attending the preached Word. If we preach the same miracle-working Jesus whom Philip preached in Acts 8, the multitudes will still be made to wonder and believe, beholding the miracles that are wrought. If we are endued with the same spirit of power that filled Paul on the Isle of Melita in Acts 28, we will still see sinners turning to Christ and the sick healed, even as did this man of God. The same resultant signs and wonders will attend our ministry.

The Word of God, therefore, while lifting our hope mountain high as we read of the power of Jesus to heal the bodies as well as the souls of His people, gives us no occasion to teach that this power was but a transitory, flitting ray of sunshine, shining for a moment through the gloom and then departing, leaving us in greater darkness than as though we had not seen the light. While the Bible gives every encouragement of healing through Jesus (see, for example, Isaiah 53; Psalm 103; Matthew 8:18; Mark 16:18; James. 5:14), there is not a verse of Scripture that would indicate that Christ had now closed this door of hope and healing for suffering bodies to the knockings of His children.

The reason that so many have tried to hide behind Paul's thorn in the flesh (see 2 Corinthians 12:7–10)—though they have never been able to quite decide just what it was, and although the conjecture runs all the way from poor eyesight or stammering utterance to an unbelieving wife—is because they feel some explanation should be made for the lack of this power in the church today. Ministers have sometimes sat up all night during our meetings searching the Bible and reading between the lines in the hope of finding some verse or passage suggesting that divine healing had been done away with, thus forming an alibi and allowing them to explain to their flock the failure to teach this truth or to pray for the healing of the sick.

What Is the Difference Between Divine Healing and Christian Science?

Christian Science teaches that there is no sin and no sickness, that such thoughts are error and that all that is needed is the power of mind over matter to overcome. Their foundation for this statement is based upon the Scriptures that tell us that without God, nothing was made that has been made (see John 1:3), and that God saw everything that He had made and, behold, it was very good (see Genesis 1:31). Because, they say, there was nothing made except that which God made, and because He made neither sin nor sickness, there is therefore no such thing as sin or sickness. Train your mind to believe this, disregard sickness and pain, exert your mind to correct this error, and all is well.

This, however, is not the teaching of the Bible. Sin and sickness were brought into the world through the fall, when Satan entered the garden of Eden in the form of a serpent, deceived Eve, and brought in, through disobedience to God, the curse of sin, suffering, thorns, and thistles.

The Bible teaches us that there is not only such a thing as sin but that it is exceedingly sinful, and that no amount of correct thinking or turning over of new leaves or cultivation of self-righteousness can cleanse us from its stain. We are told that there is but one remission of sin, and that it is the shed blood of Jesus Christ, the only begotten Son of the Father.

The Bible tells us that there is such a thing as sickness, and that Jesus "*took our infirmities, and bare our sicknesses*" (Matthew 8:17). In its discussion of the provision for our healing and deliverance, the Word of God does not tell us to "call in a practitioner" who will help us concentrate the power of mind over matter by telling us that we are not sick and that there is no such thing as sickness or pain, and then charge for treatment. Rather, it says:

> If there are any sick among you, let them call for the elders of the church and let them pray over him, anointing with oil in the name of the Lord, and the prayer of faith shall save the sick and the Lord shall raise him up, and if he have committed sins, they shall be forgiven him.
>
> (James 5:14–15)

Will Turning to Medical Aid Keep Me from Heaven?

No, it is sin that bars us out of heaven. Divine healing is not a law; it is a blessed privilege. Divine healing is like a beautiful, flowing well of cool, crystal water on a hot and dusty day. You do not *have* to drink it. You can drink the brackish water of the pond or go thirsty, if you would rather. But the well is right here, and the water is cool, refreshing, and free, and here is the dipper of believing prayer with which to draw, hanging right by the well.

Divine healing is like a beautiful shade tree in a weary land or an oasis in the wilderness. There is no law forbidding you to walk in the broiling sun at noonday, but it is your privilege to rest beneath the shadow and healing wings of the Almighty. Thousands who have found the arm of flesh to fail them have now come to lean hard upon Jesus as their all in all for body, soul, and spirit.

Coming to Christ for divine healing is like taking your watch to a watch-maker for repairs. You could take it to a blacksmith, of course, or to an automobile mechanic, and he might clumsily do his very best for you; but, after all, it would only be a second best. You have the privilege of taking the watch, with its delicate mechanism, to the very one who made it and knows just how to repair it.

When we bought our automobile, a salesman kindly said to us, "Now, any time your car needs fixing up or servicing, we will be glad to have you come right in. We will fix it free of charge. This is our own make of car, we understand it thoroughly, and our system of service is included for a certain length of time without any additional cost to you." Now, of course, there was no law to hinder us from taking the car to some other garage, where we would pay a large sum for service and perhaps find a mechanic who knew more about a Ford than he did about the mechanism of an Oldsmobile. But a few weeks later, when some adjustments were needed, we were glad to avail ourselves of the privilege of going freely to the people who had made the car and having it there adjusted and made perfectly fit again.

So it is with our blessed Lord. It is He who made us, not we ourselves. If you would prefer an earthly physician to the Great Physician, or feel that you could trust him more, then go to him. But it is your blessed *privilege* to come to the Lord who made us, who understands our frame and knows just how to heal us without pain or suffering.

What Is Your Attitude Toward the Medical Fraternity?

"Do you fight the doctoral?" we are sometimes asked. Not at all. Some of our most blessed Christian friends and brethren are in the medical profession, but the very best of them have told us that they could only do just so much with their powders and pills and that the Lord must do the rest. Though they may be clever with their scapular and knife, there comes a day when they must say, "I can do no more; you will have to look to a higher power. Only God can help you now." We have known doctors who have much more confidence in God than in their medicines and who kneel and pray with their patients, seeing Christ conquer where they have failed.

The one is natural, the other supernatural. The one is of man, the other is of God, who made heaven and earth and all that is in them.

The laws of our country have made it almost impossible for one to die without medical advice being called in, so that a death certificate may be given. We sometimes hear, in reproachful terms, "Oh, there's Mr. So-and-so. He trusted the Lord, refused medical aid, and lay right there and died." But do you know, with all due courtesy to the medical profession, that dying a natural death is not such a terrible thing, after all, when compared with the suffering that we have seen people endure under surgical and medical treatment?

Surely, doctors should be the last ones to oppose the power of Christ to heal the sick. Blind people have come into our meetings whose eyes had been put out through the mistake of a physician who dropped some acid into the eye instead of eye water. One man, in Dallas, Texas, declared that while he cried aloud with almost unendurable agony, his eye had bulged from his head (after the mistake had been made) and burst; the other went out from sympathy.

A lady in Colorado groped her blind way to the front and told a similar story. She had suffered from weak eyes and had gone for treatment. By some mistake, the physician put something into her eyes that burned like liquid fire, and in five minutes, she said, the sight was gone. The liquid had eaten right through the lens and into the pupil before it could be gotten out.

We have met people who suffered agony, in whose abdomen a roll of antiseptic gauze had been sewn up by mistake. No, I do not think the medical profession, with all their splendid hospitals and sanitariums, should oppose healing through prayer to the blessed Lord Jesus. I never heard of Him making a mistake such as these just mentioned. Have you?

A man in San Jose, California, came into the meetings for prayer, whose toes had all been amputated because of gangrene, which had set in as a result of putting a much-advertised remedy on a corn. And, oh, the number of dope victims who have wept and mourned at our altars with shattered nerves and broken bodies, having become drug addicts through having taken constant hypodermic injections during an illness following operation. Doctors were now unable to break the chains or, outside of drugs, give their patients rest and sleep, without which they would go insane. But, bless the Lord! Jesus broke the fetter and set them free.

Splendid physicians and surgeons have sat with us on the platform in our meetings, have brought patients for prayer, and have written letters praising God that He had accomplished that which their skill and power could not do.

Doctors, hospitals, and sanitariums, with their wonderful facilities, are just the thing for those who have need of them or have not the living faith in Jesus' power to make them whole. But we who believe do claim the God-given privilege of praying to our Lord for healing, thus escaping the knife and the pain.

Then, too, there are so many for whom the doctors can do no more or who are too poor to afford specialists and tremendous doctor bills. Take, for instance, Mrs. Sisson's little baby, who was healed of two hundred sores.

This sick little baby was brought in the arms of his mother at the close of service in Denver, Colorado. She had braved the crowds for hours with this tiny, pale, and wasted mite of humanity clasped to her breast. Her own face, white and haggard, plainly bespoke her anxiety and suffering for the little one. At last, she had almost reached the steps, but there was even yet a large, tightly packed crowd between herself and the platform.

"Oh God," she whispered, "if I can only get my baby through! If the sister can only take my baby in her arms and breathe a prayer, I know he would be healed of this terrible affliction! Oh, God! Oh, God!" As we turned to leave the platform after hours and hours of steady prayer (expecting to go into another room, where the crippled and bedridden were awaiting us), our eyes were irresistibly drawn to those of that dear mother. Dark and troubled, framed in a brave white face, they flashed their message. But how could we stop now? There were thousands of others who were also waiting! Then it was that, with instinctive appeal of one mother heart to another, she unfolded the baby from her breast, lifted him high above the heads of the people, and held him out to me. Involuntarily, my mother arms shot out to take him. The crowd parted to let her through, and the child was in my arms.

"Just what is this disease, Mother dear? Don't cry so hard! Jesus will heal the little lamb," I encouraged.

"Sister, it is virulent eczema; had it ever since he was four weeks old, as many as two hundred sores have eaten their way into that little form at one time. Every time I dress Baby, the blood runs from the little body. And, oh sister, he is so brave—he tries so hard not to cry," she choked; "just holds his breath and shudders."

"There, there, Mother dear. Forget that frightful nightmare of seeing Baby suffer what you would have borne for him a thousand times if you could. Jesus bore that pain for you and Baby, too, dear. He will help you."

"Oh, I know it! I know it! I know He will just now."

Anointing the baby with oil, I pressed him close and prayed earnestly; as I returned him to the young mother, she dried her tears, and the sunshine of her smile suddenly revealed the beauty of her face before these months of sleeplessness and suffering had blanched her cheeks.

She took her baby and departed but returned a few days later to testify at a mammoth children's service. She declared that her baby was well, and, indeed, his flesh looked perfectly whole.

Pressed on every hand that morning, with some five thousand children, sick and well, we could not stop to question her. But the next morning, waking early, I jumped up and into my automobile (a beautiful Oldsmobile sedan that the Denver Olds Company loaned me during the revival) and went in search of the little mother to hear the rest of the story.

Out and out I went, beyond the suburbs of the city, and then over some very bumpy roads to Downing in search of her number.

"Why, that must be it over there," I puzzled, "and yet it's so tiny. Is it a house at all?" A little dollhouse of a place it was, about as big as one ordinary room. But it wore a fresh green coat of paint and a bumble little window box made from four boards, in which struggled some tiny plants. "Why, I believe it's the smallest, humblest, and yet the neatest little house in Denver!" I exclaimed.

Suddenly, having heard the motor and auto horn, Mrs. Sisson was at the door, the baby in her arms. How she loved that frail, little life! In a moment, she was at the car. "Oh, Sister! I am so happy! I'm singing all the day long. My baby is all well. Instead of some two hundred sores ranging from the size of a pin head to large open holes, my baby's flesh is sound and whole.

"When I came home from meeting, he slept like a log. No itching or burning at all! When I gave him his bath the next morning, I found that every sore, except four of the deepest ones, had disappeared, and this morning, in the baby's bathtub, the last scab of the last four sores fell off. My baby is well! Thank God! Thank God! Christ has visited our little home."

Little home, indeed! It was little more in size than a sweet bird's nest. These dear people must be very poor and struggling hard. What this must mean to them. *Why, this is the very home of all others Christ would have surely visited in Denver*, I mused. And surely He had visited it, this blessed Man of Galilee; surely His own dear feet had crossed the threshold of that door, bringing the balm of Gilead to a fevered, tossing babe and a mother's bleeding heart, and lighted the lamp of salvation and blessing on the altar of that home.

"Yes," she replied to my question, "I took him to the doctor, and he did the best he could for baby, but the doctor finally told me that my baby had grown so bad, I would have to take him to a specialist in the city and have each sore treated every day. But"—here a brave, twisted little smile told the struggle— "my husband is only a substitute in the post office, you know. Some weeks he brings home ten dollars; sometimes ten dollars in two weeks. It takes some planning to keep soul and body together and clothes and doctor bills. So, even though Baby bled and suffered so cruelly each time I changed or bathed him, I couldn't afford the specialist but walked the floor and wept.

"Then one day came the ray of light! We had heard of a revival meeting being held in town but did not give it much thought until word came that Jesus was healing the sick today, just as He did in olden days.

"Here was my door of hope, for if it was true that Jesus still healed the sick, I had found a *specialist* where I could take my baby free of charge. Had He not said: 'Suffer the little children to come'? Was not this salvation and healing without money and without price?

"That day, I just dressed and wrapped up my poor baby and went. The rest you know. Only look, Sister; see how his little arms are filling out! He is eating everything and putting on weight. Oh, I'm so happy!"

And so was I, as I backed the car to turn and drive away. I wiped the tears from my eyes, to be able to see those ruts better, for the road was full of them, and wiped them again several times on the way to town.

"Oh Lord, I'd rather have You visit that tiny box of a house, with its coat of fresh green paint, its brave little window box, and poor young family, than the richest mansion in the land," I whispered, and drove back into a day brimful of duty and demands.

During the months that have elapsed, the mother writes that her baby is well and has gained pounds in weight, and that her husband has secured a permanent position in the post office at a splendid salary. Surely, none could object to the joy of salvation and healing being brought to that humble home.

What Should Be the Attitude of the Church Toward Divine Healing?

There is only one way in which to rightfully answer this question, and that is from the Word of God. The attitude taken by the church today should be identical to that taken by the children of God in Bible days. It should be the attitude that Moses took when the Lord spoke to him concerning the children of Israel:

*If thou wilt diligently hearken to the voice of the LORD thy God, and wilt
do that which is right in his sight, and wilt give ear to his commandments,
and keep all his statutes, I will put none of the diseases upon thee, which I
have brought upon the Egyptians; for I am the LORD that healeth thee.*

(Exodus 15:26)

Moses took the Lord literally at His word, and when sickness and plague
did come, as a direct result of sin and disobedience on the part of his people,
he cried to the Lord, and the plague was stayed. When his sister, Miriam, was
stricken with leprosy, he knew just how to pray the prayer of faith—*"Heal
her now, O God, I beseech thee"* (Numbers 12:13)—and it was done even as he
asked.

The attitude of the church toward divine healing should be that of Elijah
toward the widow's son and of Elisha toward the Shunammite's son and toward
Naaman the leper—that of faith and power in prayer to the living God.

But such miracle-working faith can be had from God only through a very
close walk with Jesus. It does not mix well with concerts, plays, moving pictures in the parish house, bridge parties, and smokers.

The attitude of the church toward divine healing should be the attitude of
David when he cried:

*Bless the LORD, O my soul: and all that is within me, bless his holy name.
Bless the LORD, O my soul, and forget not all his benefits: Who forgiveth
all thine iniquities; who healeth all thy diseases; who redeemeth thy life
from destruction; who crowneth thee with lovingkindness and tender
mercies.* (Psalm 103:1–4)

It should be the attitude of Isaiah, when he said of Christ, *"He was
wounded for our transgressions, he was bruised for our iniquities: the chastise-
ment of our peace was upon him; and with his stripes we are healed"* (Isaiah
53:5).

The attitude of the church toward divine healing should be the attitude
of the Master, who went about doing good and delivering those that were
oppressed of the devil; who said, *"As ye go, preach, saying, The kingdom of*

heaven is at hand. Heal the sick, cleanse the leper, raise the dead, cast out devils: freely ye have received, freely give" (Matthew 10:7–8); and who also gave the Great Commission: "*Go ye into all the world and preach the gospel to every creature…and these signs shall follow them that believe; In my name they shall cast out devils…they shall lay hands on the sick, and they shall recover*" (Mark 16:15, 17–18).

Ours should be the attitude of the early church, of whom we read, "*And they went forth, and preached every where, the Lord working with them, and confirming the word with signs following*" (Mark 16:20).

It should be the same attitude of Peter, when he said, "*Silver and gold have I none; but such as I have give I thee: In the name of Jesus Christ of Nazareth rise up and walk*" (Acts 3:6). When Peter had spoken these words,

> *he took him by the right hand, and lifted him up: and immediately his feet and ankle bones received strength. And he leaping up stood, and walked, and entered with them into the temple, walking, and leaping, and praising God.*　　　　　　　　　　　　　　　　　　　　　　　(Acts 3:7–8)

Ours should be the attitude of the early church when encompassed on every hand by worldliness, sin, and unbelief. The disciples knew the secret of awaking interest, silencing unbelief, and tearing down the strongholds of doubt and indifference, and cried:

> *And now, Lord, behold their threats: and grant unto thy servants, that with all boldness they may speak thy word. By stretching forth thine hand to heal; and that signs and wonders may be done by the name of thy holy child Jesus. And when they had prayed, the place was shaken where they were assembled together; and they were all filled with the Holy Ghost, and they spake the word of God with boldness.*　　　　　(Acts 4:29–31)

Our attitude should be that of Peter when, in Acts 5, by the power of Jesus, the healing of the sick, and the working of signs and wonders through his prayer, the entire country was shaken for miles around; or Philip, when, in Acts 8, a whole city was turned to Christ because they saw and heard "*the miracles which he did*" (verse 6); or James, when he left explicit directions for the healing of the sick through the prayer of faith. (See James 5:13–15.) It should be the attitude of John Wesley when he prayed successfully for the healing of the sick and saw many diseases among the people, and even the lameness of his horse, healed in answer to prayer.

Is There a Grave Danger of the Church or Individuals Being Puffed Up and Exalted by the Power Manifested in Their Midst?

The danger to be feared from this source is not nearly as great as one would at first suppose. The Lord has some very effective methods of keeping His children humble today, even as He had in the Bible days.

Take, for instance, the story of the most wonderful revival of healing on record. It is found in the fifth chapter of Acts. We read that:

> *By the hands of the apostles were many signs and wonders wrought among the people…and believers were the more added to the Lord, multitudes both of men and women. Insomuch that they brought forth the sick into the streets, and laid them on beds and couches, that at least the shadow of Peter passing by might overshadow some of them. There came also a multitude out of the cities round about unto Jerusalem, bringing sick folks, and them which were vexed with unclean spirits: and they were healed every one.*
> (Acts 5:12, 14–16)

How wonderful! One would expect the entire city to be in love with Peter and his gospel. They were, too. That is, almost all of them.

If there ever was any likelihood of Peter getting puffed up, it was on this day, but the Lord had a strong preventative ready. Opposition was raised up, not from among the common people who heard him gladly, but from the most unexpected quarter you could have imagined: the clergy!

"Here! Here! These people are taking away all our crowds, emptying our synagogues, and stirring up altogether too much excitement!" And so we read, starting in the very next verse:

Then the high priest rose up, and all they that were with him…and were filled with indignation, and laid their hands upon the apostles, and put them in the common prison. But the angel of the Lord by night opened the prison doors, and brought them forth, and said, Go, stand and speak in the temple to the people all the words of this life. (Acts 5:17–20)

They were obedient to the heavenly vision, but before the day was over, they were called to stand before the council:

When they had called the apostles, and beaten them, they commanded that they should not speak in the name of Jesus, and let them go. And they departed from the presence of the council, rejoicing that they were counted worthy to suffer shame for his name. And daily in the temple, and in every house, they ceased not to teach and preach Jesus Christ. (Acts 5:40–42)

History repeats itself in this, as in other things, and often the only opposition (in sight, at least) comes from this, the least expected quarter.

Take again the experience of Paul and Barnabas in the fourteenth chapter of Acts, after the healing of the man of Lystra.

In a loud voice, seeing that the man had faith, Paul had commanded him to stand upright on his feet. The man, who had never walked in all his life, leaped and walked, and…

When the people saw what Paul had done, they lifted up their voices, saying in the speech of Lycaonia, The gods are come down to us in the likeness of men. And they called Barnabas, Jupiter; and Paul, Mercurius, because he was the chief speaker. Then the priest of Jupiter, which was before their city, brought oxen and garlands unto the gates, and would have done a sacrifice with the people. Which when the apostles, Barnabas and Paul, heard of, they rent their clothes, and ran among the people, crying out, And saying, Sirs, why do ye these things? We also are men of like passions with you, and preach unto you that ye should turn from these vanities unto the living God, which made heaven, and earth, and the sea, and all things that are therein: And with these sayings scarce restrained they the people, that they had not done sacrifice unto them. (Acts 14:11–18)

If ever Paul and Barnabas had reason to be puffed up, it was in this city, where multitudes were ready to fall down and worship at their feet. Then, though they remained humble and gave the honor to Jesus, the Lord saw fit to send along the great preventative after all this praise and commendation of the people. And the next verses show the fickleness and changeableness of the multitudes:

> And there came thither certain Jews from Antioch and Iconium, who persuaded the people, and, having stoned Paul, drew him out of the city, supposing he had been dead. Howbeit, as the disciples stood round about him, he rose up and came into the city: and the next day he departed with Barnabas to Derbe. (Acts 14:19–20)

And so it is through the whole book—fire and water are equally mixed—so that the children of the Lord do not become puffed up or vainglorious, and so that God may have all the honor and praise, for His glory He will not give to another. (See Isaiah 42:8.)

There is nothing to be puffed up over in the praise and fawning adulation of the crowds, for those who today cry "Hosannah" and scatter palm branches may be the very ones who will tomorrow cry, "Crucify." *"God forbid that I should glory, save in the cross of our Lord Jesus Christ, by whom the world is crucified unto me, and I unto the world"* (Galatians 6:14).

Do not expect that the path, seemingly so strewn with roses, will be without a thorn. *"It is enough for the disciple that he be as his master, and the servant as his lord. If they have called the master of the house Beelzebub, how much more shall they call them of his household?"* (Matthew 10:25).

Who Can Pray for the Sick and Afflicted?

The afflicted. The Lord has so conveniently arranged the availability of His power and suited it to our helplessness and need that, should we be left alone in the wastes of the desert or far away on the country farm, in need of the Great Physician but with no one to pray for us, we can still be healed by His gracious power.

*"Is any among you afflicted? Let **him** [the afflicted one] pray. Is any merry? Let him sing psalms"* (James 5:13). The little mother wakened in the night by the choking of her little babe with a sudden attack of croup may live so close to Jesus that she can reach out her hand in faith, lay it upon the afflicted throat, pray the prayer of faith, and claim instant relief and healing.

It is doubtful whether there is a more helpless moment in a mother's life than this, when she is far away in the country, isolated from medical help or friends. Is this not a practical religion, wherein our Savior, the Great Physician, is ever within call for those who believe in His name and walk uprightly?

The elders. Again, if the pastor is busy or unavailable, we are told to call for the elders of the church and let them pray over us, anointing with oil in the name of the Lord, and that the prayer of faith will heal the sick, and the Lord will raise him up. (See James 5:14–15.)

To be truly biblical in our selection of elders, we should select men who are filled with faith and the power of the Holy Ghost, whose hearts and minds are stayed on God. It would be a terrible thing if a hurry-up call were sent for the elders, and one had to be brought from the pool hall, another from the theater, another from the club, and another from the card table. How could they be in the Spirit of God to pray the prayer of faith and claim the holy promise?

The minister of the gospel, the evangelist, the pastor, and any earnest Christian should all be able to pray the prayer of faith for the healing of the sick, whether they have received the "gift of healing" or not. *"Pray one for another, that ye may be healed"* (James 5:16). The minister and the elder must walk close to God and be men whose sober, godly, Spirit-filled lives enable them to pray the prayer of faith.

What Is the Difference Between the Prayer of Faith and the Gifts of Healing?

The prayer of faith, as we understand it, is just what its name indicates—a prayer of faith: "Oh Lord, Your Word is true. Your promises are yes and amen to everyone who believes. And now, dear Jesus, we bring our brother or sister in the arms of faith to Your throne. Be pleased to lay Your hand in healing and blessing upon this afflicted one, that he/she may be made whole from this very hour."

The gifts of healing, coming as a special unction from God, at special times, in special cases, usually according to the tide of faith, cry: "In the name of Jesus Christ of Nazareth, be made whole! Rise up and walk!" (See Acts 3:6.) This gift commands the blind eyes to be opened and the deaf ears to be unstopped. It is as though the power and authority of God, through the Holy Spirit, descends upon and envelops one for the time being, even as the mantle of Elijah fell upon and clothed Elisha.

Just What Benefits to the Church Are Derived from Divine Healing?

The practical benefits that the church derives from the healing of the sick are substantial and manifold.

1. It awakens the interest of entire communities and convinces infidels who have heretofore cried, "Where is your God?" Like the dynamic challenge of Elijah, "*The God that answereth by fire, let him be God!*" (1 Kings 18:24), it brings down the power from heaven.

2. It draws multitudes unto Jesus, causing them to repent and make Him their Savior, who were previously cold and indifferent to revivals or religion of any kind. The very act of preparing for healing, as set forth in this volume, leads the petitioner to Calvary's fountain and places him upon the altar of consecration.

3. It is a death blow to indifference and sets thousands to the unaccustomed task of reading the Bible to see whether these things are so.

4. It packs the church that has been previously only occasionally filled by some gigantic entertainment or special effort, and it gives you the opportunity to pour the blessed gospel into open, receptive hearts.

5. It is God's answer to Christian Science, and, as such, it will help you win back the members you have lost when they turned to the only church they could find that expressed any interest in the physical welfare of the people.

6. It will benefit the blind in that, when healed, they can read the Bible; the deaf in that they can hear the preached Word; the lame knees in that they can again kneel in prayer to the Lord Jesus. It will stimulate your own faith insomuch that you can see and feel the hand of the Lord working with you, confirming the Word with signs following.

May It Not Be That Much of Our Sickness Is Sent from the Hand of the Lord to Make Us Better Christians or to Keep Us from Wandering Away?

This is an old and often-advanced theory, but it is without foundation in the Word of God. The thought of our tender, sympathizing Jesus planting within His children cruel cancers to burn and gnaw and eat their way into the very heart of the sufferer, or paralysis to the limbs of little children so that they can run and play no more, or blindness to the eyes of the father so that he can no more earn his daily bread, or venereal diseases to children so that they will be made imbecile and crippled, is hideous and to not be thought of.

This is not the work of our Lord but of the archfiend Satan, whose work Jesus came to destroy. When the Lord made the world, it was pure, innocent, and free from sin and sickness. It was the devil who sowed these seeds, but there is deliverance through the triune God for body, soul, and spirit. "Well, but there is Brother Smith; he is such a holy man. He has been seated patiently in that chair for over twenty-five years! Do you not suppose that the Lord sent that stroke of paralysis to him? Who knows but that he might have been a wicked sinner or a backslider, had this blow never come?"

"Indeed, Brother Smith is a dear, precious Christian, a striking example of patience, fortitude, and strength, but I cannot believe that God tied him to that chair for twenty-five years for fear he might run away from Him and become a sinner. It is not enforced service or conscription our Lord demands but freewill enlistment. If, as you say, the Lord sends diseases, creates suffering bodies and sorrowing homes, to make us better Christians, why not get some vials of germs—diphtheria, TB, infantile paralysis, and the like—from the laboratories and scatter them over the congregation to make us all more patient and Christlike? If a little is good, would not more be better?

Is It Then a Sin to Be Sick?

No. Some of the godliest men and women you know are saints of the Most High and will soon be over on the glory side. And there are some for whom, for some reason, deliverance does not seem to come; and, as we have already said, divine healing is not a law but a blessed privilege for those who can press through and touch the Master's garment.

Is It Wise to Teach Our People to Endure with Meekness the Chastisement as Something Sent to Teach Us Patience?

This question brings a case of little Miss J., of Los Angeles, to mind. For some twenty years, the consolation of the church to her had been along this very line. "This is your cross," she was told. "Bear it patiently and with submission."

Poor, frail little body, she had quivered under the surgeon's knife again and again, but the old trouble would still return. After being confined to her bed for eighteen months after the last abdominal operation, the shades had been kept down because of her nervous prostration and suffering. She heard, through a friend, of the meetings and of the power of Christ to heal the sick.

She was almost ready for another operation to be performed but grasped the idea of deliverance through Christ as a dying man might clutch a straw, only this wasn't a straw. It was, to her, a life buoy firm and strong and sure. She laid hold upon it and held it fast, determined to arise, attend the meetings, and have prayer offered for her healing.

Her dear pastor came and talked to her sweetly again about being patient and submissive to the will of God, but she had tried that way for so many years, and had suffered so many torturous crucifixions worse than death, that it seemed as though she just could not go through it all again. And though he at last told her there was nothing to divine healing and that he disapproved of her going to the meeting for prayer, Miss J., herself the daughter of a Presbyterian minister, pressed in and claimed the promise.

She was wheeled into the meeting in a rolling chair. Healed, she shouted the praises of the Lord and, in a short space of time, was testifying and praying for sinners at the altar. Tests came later, but the Lord took her through triumphantly, making her a shining light and a winner of many souls.

The dear minister seemed to be put out and almost angry when the sister returned home, discharged her nurse, and sang and rejoiced in the newfound strength and the baptism of the Holy Spirit. But I don't see why he should be angry. Do you?

Do You Hold the Theory That We Can Live Forever in This Mortal Body?

Not at all. A man's years will be threescore and ten in the plan of our heavenly Father. But there is *protection* for the saints of God, for…

He shall cover thee with his feathers, and under his wing shalt thou trust: his truth shall be thy shield and buckler. Thou shalt not be afraid for the terror by night; nor for the arrow that flieth by day; nor for the pestilence that walketh in darkness; nor for the destruction that wasteth at noonday. A thousand shall fall at thy side, and ten thousand at thy right hand; but it shall not come nigh thee. Only with thine eyes shalt thou behold and see the reward of the wicked. Because thou hast made the LORD, which is my refuge, even the Most High, thy habitation. There shall no evil befall thee, neither shall any plague come nigh thy dwelling. For he shall give his angels charge over thee, to keep thee in all thy ways.…Because he hath set his love upon me, therefore will I deliver him. I will set him on high, because he hath known my name. He shall call upon me, and I will answer him: I will be with him in trouble; I will deliver him, and honor him. With long life will I satisfy him, and shew him my salvation. (Psalm 91:4–11, 14–16)

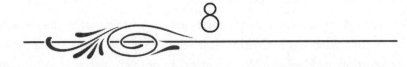

GOD'S PATTERN FOR A MODEL REVIVAL

The biblical pattern for a model revival is given us in the eighth chapter of the book of Acts. This revival reaches, as all model revivals should, in three directions, touching body, soul, and spirit. Its teachings ring forth clearly, declaring a triune God for a triune man. Its methods are simple, practical, powerful, and effective in bringing thousands to Christ.

Its threefold theme and presentation of Jesus Christ embraces salvation, divine healing, and the baptism of the Holy Spirit; a revival that fails to teach and see results along these three lines is more or less a failure and falls short of the biblical pattern of a model revival.

There were no great committee promotion boards or earthly organizations to assist Philip. There were no mammoth preparations made. In fact, a revival and a turning to Jesus Christ was farthest from the minds of the people of that city, and yet, the logical, Spirit-filled, Christ-exalting preaching of one man, accompanied by the demonstration and power of the Holy Spirit that backed up the Word, brought about such a soul-shaking revival that it turned the city upside down; caused the castles of doubt, superstition, and sin to fall crumbling to the dust; and swept thousands into the kingdom.

There is nothing mysterious, hidden, or beyond spiritual comprehension in the methods Philip used in bringing it about. He had the God-given pattern of the Word. He laid it on the whole cloth of that city and, with the scissors of the Holy Spirit, cut true to form.

We are told what steps led up to the revival, what brought the crowds of people together, what made them believe when they did come, and what happened when they did believe. We are given a complete pattern. Why should we not, therefore, pray to God for such a model revival of old-time power today as shook Samaria in the days of old?

Preparation

One of the great reasons why the efforts of so many ministers and evangelists fail is either that their own hearts have never been prepared or that they have lost their first love, with the result that their faith has grown dull and cloudy. Philip was prepared in heart, faith, and message.

He had a positive knowledge and testimony as to the definite time and place when he first saw the Christ whom he preached. Jesus had *found* him and spoken those two tender, thrilling words: *"Follow me"* (John 1:43). There and then, Philip had become not only a follower of the Christ but an active soulwinner. We read in the very next verse that Philip *found* Nathaniel, whom he told that he had *found* the Christ.

To be a successful evangelist or soulwinner, we, too, must have a definite testimony of "know-so" salvation, a definite knowledge of sins forgiven and of the hour when we were born again and all things became new.

Philip had had an intimate walk and relationship with Jesus. For three years, he had gazed into that loving face bending over the sea of humanity that ever thronged His path. He had listened to the tenderness in the voice of the Master calling the sheep who had gone astray, teaching the multitudes the way of salvation, and gently saying to Mary Magdalene, "Thy sins, which were many, are all forgiven. Go in peace and sin no more" (see John 8:11), till his own voice and heart had caught that melting tenderness.

He had seen Christ lift the fallen and cheer the faint; he had seen Him heal the sick and make the lame to walk. He had seen the glad light, like happy dawn after a night of terror, transfigure a mother's face when her sick and crippled child had been made whole and stood upon her feet.

He had seen the indescribable joy of the blind when first they gazed upon the trees, the earth, and the flowers, till their eyes found and lingered longest on the fairest of them all, the Rose of Sharon, the Lily of the Valley, the Bright and Morning Star.

He had heard the Master say,

Go ye into the world, and preach the gospel to every creature....And these signs shall follow them that believe; In my name shall they cast out devils; they shall speak with new tongues...they shall lay hands on the sick, and they shall recover. (Mark 16:15, 17–18)

He that believeth on me, the works that I do shall he do also; and greater works than these shall he do; because I go unto my Father. (John 14:12)

He had not only beheld his crucified, resurrected Lord ascending into the heavens, but *he had tarried in the city of Jerusalem*, until, with rushing wind and tongues of flame, he was baptized with the Holy Ghost and with fire.

Thus equipped with a knowledge of Christ as his *personal Savior*; a heart filled with the *tenderness* of the Master, bleeding over humanity; an *endowment of power* of the Holy Ghost, as an equipment for service; and a mountain-high *faith* in Christ's ability and faithfulness to back up the preached Word, he went forth in His name to the city of Samaria, which was to be the scene of the coming revival.

His Text—Christ

Arriving upon the scene of action, Philip went to work in a direct, businesslike, logical way. We read, *"Then Philip went down to the city of Samaria, and preached Christ unto them"* (Acts 8:5).

He did not preach politics, social reform, community uplift, theories, or doctrinal differences, but he preached *Christ*—not a different Christ from the one who had walked the shores of Galilee, forgiving sin and healing the sick; not a limited Christ whose power had waned; nor a far-off Christ who could not hear, but the Christ whose power was just the same, a Christ who had said, *"Lo, I am with you alway, even unto the end of the world"* (Matthew 28:20).

"And preached Christ to them"—what stupendous power is held captive in those words! It is as though mighty hands had firmly caught the curtains of space and intervening years and swept them wide apart to let the glory of the present Christ shine through.

Oh, Philip, how we wish that we could have slipped softly into one of the back seats and heard you preach Christ! What did you say about Him, Philip? Did you tell of the virgin birth and the babe of Bethlehem in the manger so lowly? Did you tell of the Christ, clad in mighty power, giving light to those who sat in darkness and the shadow of death; bringing deliverance to the captive and sight to the blind; causing the deaf to hear, the lame to walk, the hungry to eat in plenty and be satisfied? Did you tell of the joy of salvation? Of the Christ who supplied each need?

Oh, I am sure that you did! And as the people listened, spellbound by the tale you told, new light, new hope, new visions came to them, flowing like a river from the fountainhead of God.

Preaching Backed Up by Signs Following

How handicapped would Philip have been, had he been obliged to preach a different Christ, a limited Christ? He would have needed to say to Samaria, "Now, dear people, while I am preaching Christ to you and telling of the things He did while on this earth, you must not expect to see them now, for the light of supernatural and miraculous demonstrations of the power of Christ is passed away with His ascension."

Somehow I do not believe that the revival would have been nearly as great and wonderful. Do you? But, praise the Lord, he knew no such handicap, and as he preached Christ unto them, he was able to say, "Come, dear sinner, come to the living Jesus now. Forsake your sin. Give Him your entire being, seek

His face, believe in Him with the whole heart, and even now He will be your Savior. He will pardon your sin-sick soul. He will heal your body. He will bear your burdens and will be your all in all."

> *And the people with one accord gave heed unto those things which Philip spake, hearing and seeing the miracles which he did. For unclean spirits, crying with loud voice, came out of many that were possessed with them; and many taken with palsies, and that were lame, were healed.*
>
> (Acts 8:6–7)

Why, how could they help taking heed when they saw and heard the miracles that were done? Notice, in this pattern for a revival, that the reason for the crowds, the attention, the believing, and the results is attributed to the fact that the people saw and heard the miracles—the signs following—the official, inimitable seal of divine sanction and approval from heaven, which followed Christ's ministry and that of Peter, Paul, and James.

"And there was great joy in the city" (Acts 8:8): joy in the heart of the mother when her blind baby saw her face for the first time. Joy in the home where there once was wrangling and wrath but where now reign the altar, family worship, and love. Joy in the hearts of the Christians when they see the answer to their prayers. Joy in the once-parched desert, now blossoming as the rose.

Philip's Method Brings Awakening and Conviction to Entire City

"But what is the good of all this?" you ask. "What is the ultimate result of these healings of the body? Will they not ultimately go down into the grave, anyway? Would it not be better to do a work for the spirit, which lives forever?"

But do you not see, dear heart, that this is just what *did* happen? The healing of the body brought the people to Christ. *"When they believed Philip preaching the things concerning the kingdom of God, and the name of Jesus Christ, they were baptized, both men and women"* (Acts 8:12).

Divine healing served as the handmaiden of the gospel. Divine healing was the turnkey who went ahead to the doors of doubting castle and swung them upon their creaking hinges so that the Son of Righteousness might enter in with healing in His wings, drive back the dominion of night, and set the prisoners of darkness free.

The very Christ whose own ministry had been so marked with His healing of the sick and who asked, *"Whether is easier, to say, Thy sins be forgiven thee; or to say, Arise, and walk?"* (Matthew 9:5), was with Philip, confirming the preached Word with signs following, and there was nothing left to do but believe.

These were not mere empty theories. These were practical, tangible facts and realities. A living Christ was being preached unto them, who had the power and the willingness to change their lives from darkness into light, to lift their burdens, to heal their sick, to banish their sin, and to clothe them with righteousness and joy.

Who could resist such a mighty Christ or withstand such a convincing argument? Not Samaria, at least—so the whole city turned to Christ.

Now we today, having our hearts cleansed by the precious, atoning blood of Jesus, having faith within us and such a baptism of Holy Spirit power as that which Philip received on the day of Pentecost, may still go forth, preaching the Word of God with boldness, and see our Christ confirm the Word with signs following, thus bringing multitudes to His feet. We should be able not only to preach about this power; we should also see it demonstrated in our midst, as Philip did in Acts 8:7, as Peter did in Acts 5:14–16, and as Paul in Acts 28:8–9, when, by this means, they turned thousands to the Christ.

What a glorious revival it was—multitudes saved, healed, and baptized in water—and great joy in the city! Even Simon the sorcerer continued with Philip and wondered while beholding the miracles and signs that were done.

The Baptism of the Holy Spirit—Crowning Glory Upon Revival

Now, many of us would have thought this revival complete, well-rounded out, and needing nothing more. The people of Samaria had a much greater experience than that of the average congregation of church members today.

And yet, though the revival had touched two phases of their lives—soul and body—there was one more thing needed, and it is this that we all need so much today: the baptism of the Holy Spirit.

> *Now when the apostles which were at Jerusalem heard that Samaria had received the word of God, they sent unto them Peter and John: who, when they were come down, prayed for them, that they might receive the Holy Ghost: (For as yet he was fallen upon none of them: only they were baptized in the name of the Lord Jesus.) Then laid they their hands on them, and they received the Holy Ghost.* (Acts 8:14–17)

A revival, in order to measure up to this scriptural model, should clearly teach and, as far as possible, help believers into the experience of the baptism of the Holy Spirit, which is an endowment of power intended to equip the Christian for service and practical soulwinning for the Master.

In recent campaigns, which have grown to such an enormous size and intensity, the writer has come to understand, as never before, how Philip, pressed on every hand with sinners seeking salvation, the sick imploring healing, and the toil of bringing the nets to land, was unable to help sweep them on to the receiving of the baptism of the Holy Spirit.

But the Lord saw to it that brethren were sent, whose sole duty it was to lay their hands upon the believers and pray for them, that they might receive the Holy Spirit.

So glorious and self-evident was the receiving of the Holy Spirit, whose incoming must surely have been identical with that received in Acts 2, 10, and 19, that Simon offered money, in hopes that he might be vested with the power to bestow such a gift, believing his fortune would be made forever, if he but had the power to impart such joy and happiness as he saw come upon the recipients of this blessed experience. This power could not be bought with money, however, but with repentance, humility, and prayer.

Here Is the Pattern for the Model Revival

The model revival reaches in three directions. It brings:

First—a model revival brings salvation and forgiveness of all sin through the precious blood of Calvary; a genuine, born-again experience; a real change of heart; and an identification with the death, burial, resurrection, and life of Jesus Christ.

Second—a model revival brings divine healing for the sick and suffering body, thus fitting the temple for strength of service.

A man, when he has purchased a dilapidated house in which he intends to reside, does not usually leave the shutters and doors hanging by one hinge, the floor boards caving in, the roof leaking, and the cellar damp and musty. He takes his hammer, screwdriver, and nails, rehangs the doors and shutters, reshingles the roof, braces the floor, and airs the damp and moldy cellar.

A good mechanic, buying a squeaky automobile with one flat tire, a rusty body, and in need of a general overhauling, does not usually run it in its ailing condition. He buys new tires, scrapes off the rust, repaints and varnishes it, tightens the bearings, oils the machinery, fills the grease pan, cleans the spark-plugs, replaces a few old parts with new, and declares his car ready for efficient service and use.

So it is with our Savior, who has redeemed us with His blood. He has purchased us, not that we might always sit around in the dilapidated condition in which our late owner, the devil, left us, but to repair, or make us over, new, that with strong bodies and a willing heart we may yield to Him our glad, glad service.

But some may say, "I would rather be as I am. I know so-and-so, one of the dearest saints, who was always ill."

All right, my dears; according to your faith, so be it unto you. If you feel that God leads you in the paths of the suffering for His name's sake, obey His voice, indeed; but many, at least, have found the Savior mending the old leaky roof, tuning up the run-down engine, and fitting the temple or the vehicle for His service.

Third—a model revival brings the baptism of the Holy Spirit. The endowment of power for service and practical, levelheaded soulwinning was needed by the people of Samaria, and it is needed for the converts of our revivals today. Power to testify, power to pray, power to glorify and exalt the adorable

Christ, power to declare the imminence of His second coming, and power to help the faint on the way.

Here is the pattern; here is the cloth. God's Word is still unchanged. How many will rise up today and, in believing faith, ask the Lord to prepare our hearts as He prepared the heart of Philip, that we may be sent forth unto the surrounding "Samarias" and crown the preaching of Christ with a model revival of the old-time, threefold power?

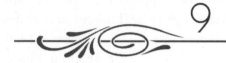

9

SOME WONDERFUL TESTIMONIES OF THOSE HEALED THROUGH PRAYER

D o the healings last? Read these testimonies from various people after several revival campaigns and healing meetings, and rejoice with us.

I had a stiff ankle of fourteen years' standing from inflammatory rheumatism. It ached and pained all the time, and I could not step on anything but I would fall. The doctors said it would never be of any use to me. On July 17, 1920, I was prayed for at the McPherson meeting in Alton and was instantly healed and never have had an ache or pain in my ankle since. Glory to Jesus and His healing power.

When I saw His power to heal, I called upon Him in the name of Jesus to take the tobacco habit away from me. I had been a slave to it for twenty-five years, chewed forty cents' worth a day, chewed so constantly that my fellow workmen called me "Tobacco Smith." I promised Jesus if He would take the habit away, I would serve Him faithfully and would never use it again. At that moment, I was caught up to heaven at the right hand of God, and when I came to myself, I knew the habit was gone. People watched me for miles around, and said, "If Tobacco Smith can quit, I will believe there is something in it." It has been the means of quite a number of my fellow workmen quitting, too.

I also praise Him that He has baptized my dear wife and me with the blessed Holy Ghost, glory to His precious name!
—*John A. Smith*
East Alton, Illinois

I wish to express my heartfelt gratitude to Jesus Christ for healing me instantly and permanently of a most terrible cancer in the lower part of my body of an internal nature, caused from bearing a son into the world. I can never express my suffering these awful years. I employed medical aid from numerous doctors and tried every known skill of doctors' science, but all to no avail. I could neither eat regularly nor sleep; I could not sit comfortably in a chair or lie in bed and get any real rest. I lost over twenty-five pounds and would cry if anyone looked at me. I spent hours in tears.

While I was in the depot at Girard, waiting to take the train for Springfield to be operated on, a telegram was handed me from my mother at Alton, Illinois. "Don't go to Springfield; come to McPherson meeting instead." I did, and God completely healed me the instant I was anointed. I have had no symptoms of the old trouble since, no aches or pains. I work hard and go out working for my Master, and I am so happy in Him!

The next day after my healing, I also had the blessed privilege of receiving the baptism and was filled with the Holy Spirit. In addition to a new body, I have a Comforter and Guide in the blessed Spirit.
—*Mrs. Lottie Inman*
Girard, Illinois

I praise Jesus for healing me and taking a fourteen-pound tumor away. The doctor said there was no hope for me without an operation. I could not keep anything in my stomach and suffered terribly. I was prayed for at the McPherson meeting last summer and afterward examined by the same doctor, and he said, "There is no trace of a tumor now." I surely praise Him with all my heart. He has since saved my husband, who was a professional wrestler and gambler, and baptized us both with the Holy Spirit. Our home is so different now, and Jesus gets all the glory. My husband was head usher at our three-day McPherson meeting here recently, and he says you couldn't have told him a year ago he would be doing that and enjoying it with all his heart. Praise our wonder-working Jesus!

—*Mrs. Elmer Cannon*
Alton, Illinois

Praise the Lord for healing me of broken arches last summer when Sister McPherson was here. I had been lame three years, the ligaments were torn loose, and the ankle bone was clear down on the bottom of the foot. Now I can run and walk and go everywhere. My husband and I have since received the baptism, and now we praise Him for what this last year has brought us.

—*Mrs. Arthur Cannon*
Alton, Illinois

I am praising God for healing me of heart trouble last July at the McPherson meeting. I have since received the baptism of the Holy Spirit and am trusting Jesus entirely for my body, never using medicine since I have found that Jesus is the same yesterday, today, and forever!

—*Mrs. James Johnson*
Alton, Illinois

I lay last year for fourteen weeks with the influenza, five weeks of that time unconscious. Then I was taken to the Westminster Hospital, where they said the flu had settled in my ankles, and I would not be able to walk. I also had eczema, and my body was all a running sore. I was carried to the McPherson meeting last summer, and God instantly healed me. Now I can walk any distance, often walking clear up to our church, a distance of about two miles. In a few weeks, I received the baptism, so now I am serving my Jesus with the strength and the power He has given me, praise His dear name!

—*Mrs. Anna Maurer*
Alton, Illinois

I praise the Lord for healing me of a running sore in my side. I was operated on, and the wound did not heal for nine months. Then I went to the tent meeting in Alton, and when Sister McPherson prayed for me, I felt the healing power go through my body; the wound closed, and it has never run a minute since then. My little boy was healed at the same time of tuberculosis. He used to be scarcely able to breathe with all the windows wide open; now he can breathe and run and play like other children. Oh, how I praise Jesus for sending Sister here to Alton.

—*Mrs. Della Henson*
North Alton, Illinois

Dear Sister: I praise God for healing me of a rupture. I was ruptured about seven years ago, and two years ago it bothered me so much, I had to wear a support, and I thought I would have to be operated on; but, praise God, He healed me last summer at the tent meeting, and I know He can heal others if they only trust in Him!

—*Mrs. Viola Guyette*
Alton, Illinois

I praise Jesus for saving me, healing me of tuberculosis, and baptizing me with His precious Spirit at the tent meeting in Alton last summer. I was brought here from Collinsville, Illinois, where I had been taking treatment for some time in a tuberculosis sanitarium. Oh, it seemed so wonderful to stand and testify and walk about and praise my Jesus during those days of the tent meeting. I want to go all the way with Him! Praise His name forever.

—*Mrs. Richard Leubbin*
Benld, Illinois

How I praise Jesus for what He has done for me—for His saving, keeping, and healing power! For seven years I had doctored for stomach and kidney trouble, trying many different doctors. I suffered constantly, could only eat bread and milk, and that with discomfort. I was prayed for at the McPherson meeting last summer, and Jesus healed me; now I can eat anything and have no pain! I praise Him because He is the same Jesus who walked the shores of Galilee. He has since baptized me with His blessed Spirit, praise His name!

—*Mrs. Fred E. Hite*
Alton, Illinois

For thirty years, I have been troubled with a most terrible spasmodic affection of the nerves. At times I have had as many as five hundred spasms of the nerves in one day, by the physician's count, but Sister McPherson prayed for me, and God wonderfully touched my body and healed me.

—*Mrs. S. Williams*
Dallas, Texas

I had stomach trouble for twenty-one years, was treated by nearly every doctor in Alton, and spent enough in doctor bills to build a church. Last summer I was saved in Sister McPherson's meeting here, and after the meetings closed, I went up to Brother Kortkamp's church and was prayed for, and the Great Physician did what no Alton doctor could do, and now I praise God for health. I gained twelve pounds in just a few weeks. In the fall, God baptized me, my wife, and three children, and this fall we are going to Auburn, Nebraska, where I will enter school to study for the ministry. Please pray for us. We want to glorify God in our lives and go all the way with Him.

—*Brother S. A. Rayborn*
Alton, Illinois

I've been sick ever since I was ten years old and have doctored for over twenty years with nearly every doctor in Alton, also with specialists. I had nervous prostration, catarrh of throat, lungs, and stomach, finally going into consumption. I never knew what it was not to be taking three or four kinds of medicine a day. Finally the doctors told me the only thing for me was to go to a different climate, though not much hope held out for that. I realized the situation and made my burial clothes, picked out the songs I wanted sung at my funeral, and wrote out the text in the back of my Bible. My clothes are still lying in the bottom of my trunk, but Sister McPherson came, and it made a change in my plans. I heard the truth of divine healing. I came up and was anointed, and I am entirely healed, not even having a symptom of the old trouble. I have gained in weight, work hard, and am serving my Savior who did such wonders for me. My husband and I have since received the baptism of the Spirit, and our home is so changed; life is worth living now, praise Jesus!

—*Mrs. Charles Goring*
Alton, Illinois

I do praise God for healing my little girl of curvature of the spine. The doctors at the clinic had told me that she must have a brace, or she would grow worse as she grew older. She was prayed for at your meeting here last summer and later was examined by the same doctors at the clinic, and they said she was all right and did not need a brace. I give Jesus all the glory. My children and I are all trusting in Jesus entirely for our healing and have taken no medicine since September. My little girl and boy, also myself, received the baptism of the Spirit, glory to Jesus! I'm so glad you came to Alton, for I was a backslider then, and now I love my Savior with all my heart.

—*Mrs. Irene Hazelwood*
Alton, Illinois

I was healed of rheumatism in July 1920, when Sister McPherson prayed for me. I had had it for two years, and it got so bad that I could not sleep for the pain. My toes and limbs would draw, and I suffered intensely. I finally became so I could not walk two blocks at a time or step up on the streetcar. I was healed completely when anointed and now can walk and run as well as ever. I give Jesus all the glory!

—*Mrs. Herman Brochies*
Upper Alton, Illinois

More than fifteen years ago, I lost my hearing from shock and cold caused by a fire that burned a building where I lived. I attended the services and heard the prayers and messages through an ear device. Here Jesus cleansed me of my sins, and when I put my trust in Him, He healed my deafness through the prayers offered up by Sister McPherson. O, I am so happy since I met and heard her pray for sinners and the sick and helpless. Praise Him! Sing more of His love!

—*Mrs. B. Winn*
St. Louis, Missouri

Dear Mrs. McPherson: I am writing you to tell you of the healing of our seven-year-old daughter, Mildred, during the meetings held by you in San Diego. She had an incurable (from a human standpoint) ear trouble, and Jesus, through your prayers, healed her. Her faith and prayers are the most beautiful I have ever heard from a child, and we can never praise Jesus enough.

—Mrs. E. S.
San Diego, California

At first, I came to Sister McPherson's meeting in St. Louis at Moolah Temple to be healed but beheld that Jesus was a living Jesus and not dead. Seeing the miracles caused me to seek salvation, and that earnestly. After making many attempts to pray my way through, I began to weep and soon found my way to the prayer room. I felt so wretched and wicked that I thought I would perish, and that I was way down in the pit with demons, but in a second, it appeared as if a shaft of lightning came out of heaven, and Jesus' hand led me safely out. I was born again and immediately received the baptism of the Holy Spirit and spoke with tongues. Even now as I write, I can feel Jesus' presence.

Of all the sins with which man's soul was blackened, I was guilty. Yes, I was chief of all sinners: cold-blooded murder, all kinds of robberies, burning houses, evil companions, vilest of habits, the worst sinner and infidel in St. Louis. Since my salvation and baptism of the Holy Spirit, it seems my old associates fear my presence, and when I touch them, they tremble. My eye afflictions are gradually disappearing as I pray. As I am able to see Jesus more, I walk closer to Him.

—Henry C. Satterwhite
St. Louis, Missouri

While attending the meetings in Moolah Temple, St. Louis, I was wonderfully healed, saved, and filled with the Holy Spirit. Through the prayers of Mrs. McPherson, I was completely healed of cancer of the stomach. Almost instantly, as she placed her hand upon my stomach, I could feel the cancer breaking loose, and I had barely time to get into privacy before the cancer passed from my body, though it was so large I had to assist in its removal. It weighed about a pound and one-quarter, and had roots ranging from one inch to six inches in length. I showed it to four persons but did not make an effort to preserve it. I was also healed of rheumatism of years' standing in my arm; I could not raise it high. Praise the Lord! I expect to serve Him the rest of my life in whatever He bids me do. My little daughter, twelve years old, was healed of deafness and blindness.

—Mrs. R. T. Gregg
St. Louis, Missouri

I wish to thank both God and you for the happy family in my home—happy in God's heart, as well as in health. I have been in bad health for three years, afflicted with a tumor, rheumatism, and nervous troubles so bad, I could not dress myself. I have been treated by six of the best physicians in the city and received no benefit. I became disgusted. When you came to our city and started the work of our Lord, I attended the meetings and became interested. I came to the altar and gave myself to Jesus Christ, heart and soul. I made two attempts to be healed with the faith and power of the Lord Jesus Christ at your hands as His disciples, failing both times to reach you because of the throng. I sent in my card and went home in prayer with my four daughters, and on the following day received the blessing. From now on, my family and I will attend church and praise God and pray as we never prayed before.

—Mrs. A. L. Ellis
St. Louis, Missouri

Seven years ago I was left in a very serious condition from child-birth. After two years and six months, I could keep up no longer; my strength left me. The doctors told me, "No hope, only an opera-tion, but don't know whether you can stand that." After the opera-tion, I was almost gone from ether pneumonia. Nine months later, I underwent another operation, and from that time, only God knows what I have suffered. I also had an attack of influenza. Doctors said I must have another operation, but I would not consent to it. The doctors of Aberdeen said, "You will come to it sooner or later; there is no other way." At Rochester, Minnesota, they said, "You cannot stand another operation, your nerves are wrecked from so much surgery. You poor woman. It's too bad,"

Later, the Lord spoke to me and said, "Trust Me, and I will heal you, and you will be well, like you were before those operations." The Lord impressed me to come to St. Louis. I was anointed and prayed for by Sister McPherson, and—glory to Jesus!—He wonder-fully touched my body and straightened that curvature of the spine. I could feel the vertebrae going into place. He healed my throat and healed my heart. He put those floating kidneys back into place and healed those adhesions. It was like an osteopath at work. I could feel the touch of His healing hand. I have no pain! Hallelujah! There is nothing too great for this wonderful Physician.

—*Mrs. J. A. Loock*
Hecla, South Dakota

I can thank the Lord for the healing of my body, as I had spinal trouble for twelve years. When I heard you were at the Hancock M. E. Church, I went down and heard your sermons, and on the heal-ing night, I went to the altar, and when you anointed and prayed for me, the pain in my back was gone, and it has not pained me since. I also praise the Lord for the baptism of the Holy Ghost.

—*Charlotte Becher*
Philadelphia, Pennsylvania

I left Allen, Oklahoma (about two hundred miles from here), and, catching a ride of about one hundred and twenty miles, walked the balance of the way, about seventy-five miles, to the meetings, and God healed my eyes after I had suffered with them about fifteen months.

—*L. L. Osborn*
Dallas, Texas

God delivered me from lung trouble. I came to the altar, got right with God, and fasted and prayed, and He healed me when Sister McPherson prayed for me. I also had a defect in my right eye, and when I got home and picked up the paper, my right eye was as clear as the left.

—*Mr. Strubel*
Clovis, New Mexico

For seventeen long years I was a sufferer with nervous asthma, and in that time, nothing was left undone that we thought would improve my health even a little bit, and I was thinking of trying an operation on my nose, but the doctors would not ensure relief even with that. Then, you came to Alton. I had often told my mother I believed I could be healed by faith in Jesus, if I had someone who was full of love and faith to pray with and for me, so when you came, I began to prepare. I had been a Christian for sixteen years, so on July 8, 1920, when I attended the Healing Service in the First Methodist Church, and you anointed me in the name of the Lord, prayer was answered. For five years, I had not been able to lie down; I could only sleep propped in a chair or propped in bed, and then, only for a few minutes at a time, and would wake choking. But praise the Lord! That awful time is over, and my last prayer at night is, May God bless dear Sister McPherson and help her in her wonderful work.

—*Miss Pearl Rayborn*
Alton, Illinois

This is my personal testimony as to the healing power of the Great Physician. Sunday evening I went up for healing, knowing that the Great Physician was healing His children, and, praise the Lord, He touched me. At the age of two years, I had diphtheria and suffered with an abscess the size of a large goose egg on the right side of my neck, close to the ear. The doctor advised my parents to scatter this abscess instead of bringing it to a head. Consequently, upon recovering from the disease, I was left afflicted with a discharging ear, the eardrum shattered, and my hearing completely gone. A few months ago, a doctor, upon an examination, said that a sac full of pus was forming close to the brain that would necessitate a very dangerous operation, and that my whole system was likewise poisoned, and that it would only be a course of time, as I would not live to be more than twenty-one years of age. Praise the Lord, I am on the road to recovery.

Since Sunday evening, the work of the Savior has been the same as told of in Bible times. That same night, my hearing, as many know, was restored after eighteen years of being entirely deaf. Monday evening, the discharge started flowing out of my head. On Tuesday, the right side of my neck was a mass of abscesses full of this corruption, which would break and refill. My ear has been continually draining since. The cords on the side of my neck are soft and at their normal size; they had been swollen and hard for years. For two days, it seemed like a raw sore was in the vicinity of my ear, and how it did burn; but that has gone now. I had not known a well day free from pain since I was a baby in my mother's arms, but glory! Glory! Glory! I am no longer a prisoner held captive to suffering, for all the pain has left my body, and I am well. The chains are broken, and, praise the Lord, I have purchased a ticket on the good old Bible line. I hope you don't get weary reading this epistle, but I just had to tell you how wonderful the love of Jesus is to me. May God bless you, Sister McPherson, and ever keep you in His arms of love; this is the wish of my young heart. Sincerely yours,

—*Irene H. Locklin*
San Diego, California

What a joy to praise the Lord! And how I love Jesus for all He has done for me! Not satisfied with shedding His precious blood on Calvary's hill to wash away my sins—glory to His name—and baptizing me with the Holy Spirit—praise Him—He, in His great love, also healed my body.

For five years, I had been suffering from a tubercular knee, which kept me in the hospital for nearly two years, and the surgeons even suggested amputation. But the Lord made me whole again, instantaneously, in the most miraculous manner, after I was prayed for by Sister McPherson. And now I can kneel down on both my knees (a thing I could not do for nearly five years) and praise my Savior. Glory! He also healed me of abdominal trouble, for which I had undergone two operations without any apparent amelioration. But the Great Surgeon did not fail. Praise His name! So, I am born again in my soul and in my body. Oh, my precious Redeemer, how I love Him; how I want to serve Him and praise Him for His great love for me!

—Mrs. Eva Quenneville
San Diego, California

I am writing this to add my testimony to all the others of those who have been healed by God through your faithful work in San Jose. I had injured some muscles in my left arm and had my arm in different casts for six months. On last Good Friday, you anointed my arm, and, true to God's Word, He healed it. I came back to Livermore and went to work the next morning using the arm same as the other, for which I certainly give God the praise.

—J. Edwards
Livermore, California

I want to give a testimony of what the Lord Jesus Christ has done for me here at Sister McPherson's meeting, August 17. I was wonderfully healed of a sagged stomach, a curved spine, and a floating kidney. My food would decay in the stomach before digesting. This came on me suddenly, and in eight months, I lost fifty pounds of flesh. Dr. Dray of the Franklin Hospital, San Francisco, has six X-ray plates of my stomach. He has been my physician for four years, so three months ago I was very ill and went to his hospital. This time, he told me I would have to have an operation to make an opening for the food to digest out and not have to make the curve.

I told him no, I would wait a while. He also said I could have the X-ray plates at any time to send my brother, who is a physician in New York. Oh, now I am so glad I did wait, for Jesus Christ has healed me forever. Now my food digests, and I can eat anything. Praise the Lord. I am now going to work for Jesus, and He will be my Healer. I have the faith. Hallelujah, praise the Lord. Amen.

—*Mrs. Ida Meister*
San Jose, California

Dear Sister: Just a few lines to let you know that we in San Diego are still keeping you in remembrance and are following your campaigns with our prayers. Oh, we do pray for you, Sister, and for the blessed outpouring of His Holy Spirit in all your meetings.

Perhaps it will be of some help to someone who is seeking more faith to know that my lung that was restored is still as good as ever, praise His loving grace. I have never had another hemorrhage since it was healed and have gained forty-six pounds, although I am working every day. The blessed Lord has given me a definite call to His service, and I expect to enter Drew Seminary to prepare for the missionary field the latter part of September.

—*James R. Flood*
San Diego, California

My Dear Sister: I must tell what my dear Master has done for me, glory to His precious name. In August, I had to have my knee-cap broken open and wired back in shape. I attended all of your most wonderful meetings, God bless you. Waiting there two weeks, seeking perfect faith, I then decided to trust it to Jesus' love instead of the hospital, for they were the cause of so much suffering. And glory! Glory! Glory! Glory to the precious name of Jesus, He took all the pain away instantly, and I could feel the pus melt away while you anointed and prayed for me; then I could feel the bones slipping back in shape. I don't know how to thank and praise my Lord and Savior enough.

I could write a book or preach a sermon on what the Lord has done for me, but I know that you are too busy to listen to me preach now. I am going out into the Lord's work soon. I can hardly hold back any longer. I must close, in Jesus' love.

—C. A. McMillan
San Jose, California

Much widespread interest was aroused during the San Diego revival by the testimony of the sailor boy [James R. Flood] whose gas mask was pierced in France so that he lay unconscious for hours, bleeding at mouth and nostrils. His officers sent him home and on to San Diego to die. X-ray photos showed the lung to be withered to the size of a goose egg and hanging to the bronchial tubes. Constant hemorrhages from the other lung made life a misery to the suffering lad. Jesus healed him in answer to prayer insomuch that the withered lung was instantly restored to life and inflated fully, and he sang aloud and shouted for joy. Our readers may ask, "Do the healings last?" The above will speak for itself.

—Editor

I praise the Lord for healing me of cancer of the breast, failing eyesight, and extreme nervousness, on the night of August 17, 1921, in San Jose, California, when I was anointed and prayed for by Mrs. McPherson.

I first began to have pain in my breast seven years ago and went to many doctors. I went to Camp Wildwood to Dr. Howard, but after some treatments, I was no better. I also went to Honolulu to a specialist, but still I was no better. The pain grew worse and worse, until the pain went down my arm, too, and I had a terrible burning in the breast and also a perfectly hard lump the size of an egg.

During this time, my eyesight was failing more and more, until I couldn't see to thread a needle, even with strong glasses. My glasses were becoming of less and less use to me, until I feared I was going blind.

I became so nervous, I could hardly bear it. I cried continually, not knowing why, and lost interest in everything and was so dis-couraged, my husband did not know what to do with me.

But my husband had great faith, too, and when the campaign started, we both went to the altar at the first meeting and re-conse-crated our lives to Jesus. Every meeting, my faith increased, until, before I went up to be prayed for, I felt the power of God through my whole body, until I thought I would fall. The pain in my breast stopped at once, and I felt the cancer swiftly melt away, and it has never returned.

Glory to Jesus! My eyesight returned at once, and I have not worn my glasses since. One of my friends doubted my healing and the next day said to me, "If you can thread this fine needle, I will be convinced that you are healed." I took this fine needle and prayed silently, "Lord, help me to thread it," and the thread went through the first try—praise the Lord!

The next day when I got up, I prayed that the Lord would increase my strength so I could get my work done and get to the meetings. The Lord gave me even more time than I had hoped for, and I did my washing, put up pickles, got all my morning work done, and was at the tent at one o'clock, ready for the meeting.

All my nervousness is gone, and I am a changed woman. Glory to Jesus! I am happier than ever before in my life and feel perfectly well. Praise the Lord forever! The cancer is entirely gone. Hallelujah.

—*Mrs. Marian N. Bishop*
San Jose, California

For twelve years, I have had attacks of loco motor ataxia, walking backward, and limbs trembling when trying to walk. At one time, the attack lasted an entire year. Doctors in various places could not understand it. They said the disease was very rare, and they have made all sorts of tests, but in vain.

When the attack came, I was not able to stand for ten days or two weeks and was filled with pain. After sitting for a while, I could not walk without going backward. Folks said I would get there quicker if I turned around. Sometimes I lost my speech during these attacks.

I also suffered much for the last four months from rheumatism, with fingers swollen so that I could not close my hands and could barely raise my arms. To add to my suffering, there was a broken bone in my ankle. When brought to the platform for prayers, I was suffering from one of my above mentioned attacks and had to be supported. I was instantly healed when prayed for, and all of the pain left my body. I could close fingers, raise my arm, and walk perfectly. Hallelujah! It is a new world to me!

—*Anna Stein Brink*
Dinuba, Tulare County, California

The bearer of this letter, Miss Embry, is one who wishes you to anoint and dedicate her to His service. I am sending by her to your mother one of my pictures, as you do not seem to have gotten the ones that were sent by mail as you asked. May He use my testimony for His glory, is my constant prayer.

A group of young folks who were working at your meetings here have been carrying on the work at the Little Normal Heights Church here, together with Brother Weyant, the pastor, and we have received some wonderful blessings from the Lord and some souls saved. Praise the Lord. We hold fasting, prayer, and tarrying meetings every Monday night, for those who are seeking the blessed baptism and spiritual and physical healing, and He has been with us wonderfully. We hope that when you find time to come to San Diego again, you will not forget the Normal Heights M. B. Church. God's blessing be with you, Sister, and with your dear mother.

—*James R. Flood*
San Diego, California

I want to give you my testimony of receiving they baptism of the Holy Spirit right away after you preached that wonderful sermon of yesterday. I felt the power coming on me, I started for my room a few blocks away, and I praised Jesus all the way to my room, under the power so mightily, I thought my feet would slip from under me and let me down on the sidewalk. But, praise God, He held me up until I got to my room, and He poured rivers of water till He filled me full and overflowing until my cup ran over, and, glory to Jesus, I spoke in tongues and rejoiced in the Lord, praising Jesus.

I am in my sixty-seventh year and am one of those old people who will testify for Jesus.

—*Mrs. J. B. Smith*
Alameda, California

I was greatly privileged in finding myself at San Jose while the meetings were in progress. I did not go there to attend the meeting. My time of vacation was at hand, and I had some business to look after. This was what led me to the city of San Jose, so I thought, but I found it was the Spirit of God.

I said I will go to the meeting on Monday night and Tuesday night and then be on my way, but Monday night was healing night. Something like fifty lame, halt, blind, deaf—many kinds of the afflicted—were healed. The blind received their sight, the deaf heard, the lame walked. Jesus was there in mighty power. I saw a deaf and dumb girl made well insomuch that she both heard and spoke. What was I, that I should withstand God? I became a seeker and tarried for the baptism of the Holy Spirit, and my new experience is wonderful.

I am very happy to witness the wonderful way Jesus is using Mrs. McPherson and the sweet spiritual pastor of the First Baptist Church, Dr. Towner. God bless them.

—*E. R. Clevenger*
Madera, California

I had been deaf in my right ear for twenty-five years and in the left ear two years, as a result of grippe and neuralgia. Specialists said the eardrum was destroyed. I heard of the meetings of Sister McPherson in San Jose, and for three weeks, I prayed to get here to be healed. Praise the Lord, He opened the way!

When our sister prayed for me, I was healed instantly. Hallelujah! As soon as these wonderful meetings so filled with the power of God are ended, I am going home to spread the glad news and work for my Lord.

—*A. B. Dean*
Atwater, California

ABOUT THE AUTHOR

Aimee Semple McPherson (1890–1944) was a woman ahead of her time. She crossed the United States with two young children in an era when women were not permitted to vote. She established an evangelistic ministry and built a large evangelistic center at a time when women were expected to marry, have children, and leave religion and other "important" pursuits to men. But God had a plan for her life that did not take into account human ways of doing things. As an evangelist who preached the gospel not only across the United States but also around the world, "Sister Aimee" incorporated the cutting-edge communications media of her day, becoming a pioneer in broadcasting the gospel on the radio.

Upon opening the doors of Angelus Temple in Los Angeles in 1923, Sister Aimee developed an extensive social ministry, feeding more than 1.5 million people during the Great Depression. She summarized her message into four major points, which she called "the Foursquare Gospel": Jesus is the Savior; Jesus is the Healer; Jesus is the Baptizer, with the Holy Spirit; and Jesus is the soon-coming King. She founded the International Church of the Foursquare Gospel, also known as The Foursquare Church, which continues to spread the Foursquare Gospel throughout the world to this day. Recently, *Time* magazine named her as one of the most influential people of the twentieth century.